SMILE YOU ARE ADDICTED

PORNOGRAPHY

MONTAZAR ALKEFAAE

Copyright © 2024 by Montazar Alkefaae

All rights are reserved, and no part of this publication may be reproduced, distributed, or transmitted in any manner, whether through photocopying, recording, or any other electronic or mechanical methods, without the explicit prior written permission of the publisher. This restriction applies to any form or means of reproduction or distribution.

Exceptions to this rule include brief quotations that may be incorporated into critical reviews, as well as certain other noncommercial uses that are allowed by copyright law. Any such usage must adhere to the specified conditions and permissions outlined by the copyright holder.

Book Design by HMDPUBLISHING

CONTENTS

INTRODUCTION 5

01. THE UNYIELDING VALUE OF WOMEN 8
Modernity 11
The industry 12

02. THE INTERNET 14
Addiction: The Devastating Impact of Pornography 16

03. THE BRAIN: A MARVEL OF CREATION 19
The Dopamine 22
Testosterone 24
Feelings of addiction 26

04. THE DEVIL 29
Victims of Pornography - From Young to Old, Women to Men 30
Lily! 31
The Impact 32
The industry 33
The art and artists of the porn industry 35
European Jews and the industry 37
Early Investments 39
Domination Continues 41
Reasons for Jewish Infiltration in the Pornography Industry .. 44

05. "YES, I CAN QUIT." 46
Free will 47
Practical Steps to Enhance Self-Awareness: 50
HCustomized Recovery Plans: 53
Benefits of Seeking and Receiving Help: 53
Overcoming Barriers to Seeking Help: 54
Steps to Setting Goals for Recovery 54

Benefits of Setting Goals for Recovery 56
Examples of Recovery Goals 57
Steps to Creating New Habits 58
Benefits of New Habits 60
Examples of New Habits 62

06. RELIGIONS AND DIVINE RELIGIONS 64
Judaism 66
Looking at Taboos and Sexual Addiction 66
Chastity and Morality 67
Christianity 68
Looking at Taboos and Sexual Addiction 68
Chastity and Morality 68
Islam 70
Hadith on Lowering One's Gaze 71
Examples from the Life of the Prophet Muhammad ... 72
Chastity in Sex 73
Hinduism 78
Pornography and Sensory Control 78
Chastity and Moral Values 78
Buddhism 78
Sikhism 79
Sabian-Mandaean 80
Other Religions 80
SUMMARY OF "SMILE, YOU ARE ADDICTED" 82
SOURCES 84
AUTHOR 100

INTRODUCTION

Imagine finding yourself unable to communicate with your partner due to impotence. It's a challenging situation, filled with feelings of inferiority and helplessness. The constant trying and failing is truly exhausting. Now, take the scenario further—imagine the possibility of separation, becoming a single parent, or a single mother. The thoughts that flood your mind are overwhelming. When you think of your children and the suffering they will endure alongside your own, the heartache becomes unbearable. You start to realize that the reason for the breakup was significant, right? What if I told you that the root cause of this turmoil is the sex videos that have consumed your attention recently? It becomes clear that you're dealing with an addiction. This is one of dozens of scenarios a porn addict may experience, starting from their teenage years and continuing into their sixties.

In our society, we often follow certain norms without questioning them. From a young age, we learn to smile, nod in agreement, and hide our true feelings to fit in. But behind these masks, we face deeper challenges, especially in our relationships. Our brains, shaped by thousands of years of evolution, help us connect with others through trust, respect, and love.

However, in today's world filled with instant gratification and constant stimulation, it's easy to lose sight of what truly matters. We are bombarded with artificial stimuli, like pornography, that promise quick pleasure but ultimately leave us feeling empty and disconnected.

Throughout history, religions like Islam, Christianity, and Judaism have emphasized the importance of strong, enduring relationships built on marriage. These faiths teach us about fidelity, loyalty, and devotion, guiding us toward deeper, more meaningful connections.

Despite these teachings, addiction can still creep into even the most sanctified unions, threatening the trust and intimacy that hold them together. The allure of pornography, the temptation of infidelity, and societal pressures can erode the foundations of our relationships.

This book aims to explore the complex world of porn addiction, uncovering its roots and offering pathways to healing and redemption. It is a journey filled with challenges, but also with hope for those ready to face their demons and embrace the truth.

As we delve into this topic, we will peel back the layers of societal expectations and examine how they impact our relationships and self-worth. We will confront the uncomfortable truths about addiction and how it distorts our desires and behaviors.

Through the stories of resilience and redemption, we will see how individuals have faced their addictions and come out stronger. These journeys serve as beacons of hope, guiding us toward healing and renewal.

As we navigate these pages, let's approach the uncomfortable truths with open hearts and minds. Only by confronting our deepest fears and insecurities can we truly break free from the chains that bind us.

Dear reader, I invite you to join me in exploring the heart of addiction. Together, we will uncover the power of authenticity in a world that often demands conformity. Through this journey, may we find the courage to embrace our true selves and build meaningful connections.

Welcome to "Smile, You Are Addicted."

CHAPTER 1:
THE UNYIELDING VALUE OF WOMEN

In the intricate tapestry of society, women stand as pillars of strength, bearing the weight of countless responsibilities with grace and resilience. They are not merely half of the population; they are the heartbeat of families, the nurturers of souls, and the architects of tomorrow.

In the traditional framework of family dynamics, men often toil tirelessly to provide for their loved ones, shouldering the burden of financial obligations. Yet, it is the woman who occupies a sacred role as the primary educator, a steadfast guide, and an endless reservoir of tenderness for all members of the household.

Indeed, she is the cornerstone upon which a healthy and harmonious family is built, weaving together the threads of love, discipline, and compassion to create a cohesive unit. Through her tireless efforts, she fosters an environment where children thrive, husbands find solace, and generations are shaped.

However, the landscape of women's roles has evolved over the centuries, shaped by the tumultuous currents of history. In bygone eras, women were shielded from the harsh realities of financial responsibility, their duties centered squarely on the hearth and home.[1] Society, in its wisdom or folly, restricted their sphere of influence, offering scant opportunities for economic independence.

Yet, the winds of change blew fiercely across Europe, sweeping aside centuries of tradition and ushering in an era of upheaval. Wars ravaged nations, famines struck with merciless force, and deadly diseases stalked the land, leaving devastation in their wake[2]. In the crucible of such adversity, women were thrust into the labor market, their hands forced by necessity rather than choice.

The industrial revolution, with its promise of progress and prosperity, proved to be a double- edged sword for women.[3] While it offered newfound opportunities for employment, it also exacted a toll on their traditional roles as caregivers and homemakers. As they entered factories and mills, they gradually drifted from their fundamental responsibilities, leaving a void in the fabric of family life. [4]

With each passing year, the once-gleaming luster of motherhood dimmed, eclipsed by the demands of the modern world. Divorce rates soared, and the ranks of single mothers swelled, bearing witness to the fraying of familial bonds and the erosion of societal norms.[5]

As we journey through the annals of history, we witness the profound impact of societal shifts on the role of women, illuminating both the triumphs and tribulations that have shaped their journey. From the confines of domesticity to the frontlines of industry, women have navigated a labyrinth of challenges with unwavering resolve, their resilience serving as a beacon of hope in the face of adversity.

Yet, amidst the tumult of progress, we must pause to reflect on the unintended consequences of such seismic shifts. The forced entry of women into the labor market, though borne of necessity, exacted a toll on the fabric of family life, disrupting age-old traditions and redefining the dynamics of domesticity.

With the rise of industrialization came a stark realization: the traditional roles of women as caregivers and homemakers were no longer sustainable[6] in the face of rapid urbanization and economic upheaval. As they stepped out of the shadows of the home and into the factories and mills, they embarked on a journey fraught with uncertainty, grappling with the delicate balance between work and family, duty and desire.

Yet, even as they embraced newfound freedoms and opportunities, women found themselves ensnared in a web of societal expectations and cultural norms. The pressure to excel in both the professional and personal spheres weighed heavily upon their shoulders, leaving many to question their worth and identity in a world that demanded perfection at every turn.

In the wake of such profound change, the fabric of family life underwent a metamorphosis, as divorce rates soared and single motherhood became increasingly common. The once-steadfast institution of marriage faltered under the weight of modernity, its foundations shaken by the shifting sands of societal norms and economic uncertainty.

Modernity

As the curtain rose on the last century, a seismic shift reverberated across the landscape of society, reshaping the contours of gender roles and redefining the very essence of womanhood. With the dawn of industrialization came newfound opportunities for women to partake in the labor market alongside their male counterparts, heralding a new era of progress and prosperity. Yet, amid the promise of economic empowerment, a shadow loomed on the horizon: the gradual erosion of modesty and chastity, as societal norms evolved to accommodate the changing tides of modernity. As women ventured into new spheres of employment, from fashion modeling to media representation, they found themselves thrust into the spotlight, their bodies commodified and objectified for the consumption of the masses.

In the land of freedom and globalization, America, the floodgates of opportunity swung wide open, beckoning women to seize their place in the sun. Yet, amidst the glittering allure of fame and fortune, a darker underbelly emerged, as establishments peddling pornographic imagery proliferated, lining their coffers with the currency of human desire.

In this brave new world, women became commodities, their worth measured not by the strength of their character or the depth of their intellect, but by the curves of their bodies and the allure of their gaze. As the demand for titillation soared, a new breed of entrepreneurs emerged, capitalizing on the insatiable appetite for carnal pleasure.

Yet, amid the clamor of commercialism, a question lingers in the air: who bears the mantle of responsibility for this descent into moral decay? Was it the hand of a single man, driven by greed and lust, or the insidious machinations of institutionalized exploitation?

As we navigate the complexities of modernity, we confront a stark reality: the commercialization of female bodies and the degradation of womanhood in the pursuit of profit. With each passing day, the lines between empowerment and exploitation blur, as women are coerced into conforming to narrow standards of beauty and sexuality.

The proliferation of pornographic imagery and the commodification of female sexuality have transformed women into mere objects of desire, stripped of their humanity and reduced to mere symbols of gratification. In the pursuit of profit, boundaries are blurred, ethics are compromised, and the dignity of women is sacrificed on the altar of consumerism.

The industry

The origins of pornographic magazines and establishments are complex and multifaceted, making it difficult to attribute their creation to a single individual or entity. However, one of the earliest known examples of pornographic publications dates back to the 19th century, with the emergence of erotic literature and explicit illustrations in various forms of media.

In the early 20th century, as advancements in printing technology made mass production more accessible, pornographic magazines began to gain popularity, catering to a growing demand for explicit content. These publications often featured nude or semi-nude images of women, alongside sexually explicit stories and advertisements for adult entertainment venues.

As the industry grew, so too did the controversies and scandals surrounding it. Many critics argued that pornographic magazines and establishments perpetuated harmful stereotypes and objectified women, contributing to the normalization of sexual exploitation and violence. There were also concerns about the impact of pornography on societal values and the erosion of traditional morals.

Opposition to the pornographic industry came from various quarters, including feminist activists, religious groups, and social reformers. These critics argued that pornography dehumanized women, promoted unhealthy attitudes towards sex, and contributed to the objectification and commodification of female bodies.

CHAPTER 2:
THE INTERNET

In the not-so-distant past, access to pornographic material was largely confined to paper publications or videos, typically relegated to discreet adult-only spaces.[1] Privacy was a prerequisite for indulging in such content, as one had to seek out physical copies or visit specialized establishments to satisfy their desires. However, the advent of the internet revolutionized the landscape of pornography, ushering in an era of unprecedented accessibility and availability.

With the rise of computer programming and the proliferation of the World Wide Web, pornographic material became just a click away for anyone with an internet connection.[2] The anonymity and convenience offered by online platforms shattered the barriers that once confined pornography to the shadows[3], making it accessible to individuals of all ages and backgrounds.

The consequences of this seismic shift were profound. Suddenly, society found itself inundated with a deluge of explicit content, bombarding unsuspecting users with images and videos that were previously confined to the fringes of society.[4] This unbridled exposure to pornography had far-reaching implications, shaping the attitudes and behaviors of a generation raised in a digital age.

As access to pornography became ubiquitous, a new generation emerged, characterized by a distorted understanding of sexuality and intimacy.[5,8] Raised in a culture saturated with explicit imagery and hypersexualized messaging, these individuals found themselves navigating uncharted territory, where the lines between fantasy and reality blurred with alarming ease.

The cultural landscape underwent a tectonic shift, as traditional values and norms gave way to a brave new world of instant gratification and moral relativism.[6] The consequences were profound, as society grappled with the fallout of a generation raised on a steady diet of pornography, struggling to reconcile the disconnect between the virtual and the real.

In shaping this emotionally distorted generation, the internet played a pivotal role, serving as both a catalyst for change and a harbinger of the challenges that lay ahead. As we confront the legacy of this digital revolution, we must reckon with the profound impact of pornography on our collective psyche[7], and work towards building a future where healthy attitudes towards sex and intimacy prevail.

Addiction: The Devastating Impact of Pornography

The allure of pornography can be intoxicating, drawing individuals into a seemingly endless cycle of consumption with devastating consequences for their mental well-being and sense of self-worth.[10] As they succumb to its seductive grip, they find themselves trapped in a downward spiral, their lives consumed by an insatiable thirst for fleeting pleasure.

The journey into addiction often begins innocently enough, with casual curiosity or fleeting interest leading individuals to explore the world of pornography. What starts as a harmless indulgence soon escalates into a full-blown obsession, as the brain becomes desensitized to the stimuli and craves increasingly extreme forms of gratification.

As addiction takes hold, the consequences become increasingly dire. Mental health deteriorates, as individuals struggle with feelings of shame, guilt, and worthlessness. Relationships suffer, as the intimacy and connection once shared with loved ones are replaced by a hollow facade of gratification.

Self-value erodes, as individuals become slaves to their desires, unable to break free from the shackles of addiction. They find themselves consumed by feelings of inadequacy and self-loathing, trapped in a vicious cycle of self-destructive behavior.

An example of the devastating impact of pornography addiction can be seen in the story of Alex, a young man who stumbled upon pornography at a vulnerable age. What started as harmless curiosity soon spiraled out of control, as Alex found himself spending hours each day consumed by explicit imagery.

As his addiction deepened, Alex's mental health deteriorated, leading to feelings of anxiety, depression, and isolation. His relationships suffered, as he withdrew from friends and family, unable to face the shame and guilt that consumed him.

Despite numerous attempts to break free from the grip of addiction, Alex found himself trapped in a cycle of despair, unable to imagine a life without pornography. It was only through intensive therapy and support from loved ones that he was able to reclaim his life and rebuild his sense of self-worth.

The story of Alex serves as a sobering reminder of the devastating impact of pornography addiction, and the importance of seeking help and support in overcoming its grip. As we confront the realities of addiction, let us remember that there is hope for recovery, and that no one is beyond redemption.

As society grapples with the pervasive influence of pornography addiction, it becomes increasingly clear that this is not merely a personal struggle, but a societal crisis with far-reaching implications. The normalization of pornography in mainstream culture, coupled with easy access through the internet, has created a perfect storm of addiction that threatens to engulf entire communities.

The mental health toll of pornography addiction cannot be overstated. Studies have shown that prolonged exposure to explicit material can lead to a host of psychological issues, including depression, anxiety, and low self-esteem. The constant bombardment of unrealistic and hypersexualized imagery distorts individuals' perceptions of themselves and others, fueling feelings of inadequacy and insecurity.

Moreover, the addictive nature of pornography hijacks the brain's reward system, leading to a cycle of compulsive behavior that is difficult to break. Like a drug, pornography provides a temporary escape from reality, offering a brief respite from the stresses and pressures of everyday life. But with each hit, the craving grows stronger, until it consumes every waking moment, leaving individuals powerless to resist its pull.

But perhaps the most insidious aspect of pornography addiction is its impact on relationships. Intimacy, trust, and communication are eroded as individuals retreat into a world of fantasy and illusion, seeking fulfillment in pixels and pixels alone. Partners feel betrayed and abandoned, left to pick up the pieces of shattered trust and broken promises.

In the face of such overwhelming challenges, it is easy to feel hopeless and powerless. But there is reason for optimism. With awareness and education, individuals can break free from the grip of addiction and reclaim their lives. Support groups, therapy, and other resources are available to help those struggling with pornography addiction find their way back to health and happiness.

CHAPTER 3:
THE BRAIN: A MARVEL OF CREATION

In the intricate tapestry of human existence, the brain stands as a marvel of creation, a wondrous network of neurons and synapses that governs our thoughts, emotions, and actions. From the moment of conception, God fashioned us in the best manner, endowing us with a complex organ capable of unparalleled feats of cognition and perception.

At the very core of our being lies the brain, a masterful creation that serves as the command center of our bodies and minds.[1] Within its vast expanse, billions of neurons fire and connect, forming intricate pathways that shape our experiences and shape our understanding of the world.[2] The brain is a testament to the divine wisdom of its creator, intricately designed to fulfill a multitude of functions with unparalleled efficiency. From regulating basic bodily functions such as breathing and heartbeat to processing complex thoughts and emotions, its capabilities are boundless.

But perhaps most remarkable of all is the brain's capacity for plasticity, the ability to adapt and change in response to experience. Throughout our lives, our brains undergo constant remodeling, rewiring themselves in response to new information and stimuli. It is this remarkable flexibility that allows us to learn, grow, and evolve as individuals, shaping our destinies and forging our paths in the world.

As we delve deeper into the mysteries of the brain, we uncover a profound truth: that we are fearfully and wonderfully made, crafted by the hand of a loving creator who fashioned us in his image. In the intricate dance of neurons and synapses, we catch a glimpse of the divine, a reminder of the boundless creativity and intelligence of our maker.

The brain's interaction with hormones is a complex and intricate dance that regulates a wide array of bodily functions, emotions, and behaviors.[3] Hormones are chemical messengers produced by various glands throughout the body, including the hypothalamus, pituitary gland, thyroid gland, adrenal glands, and reproductive organs. These hormones travel through the bloodstream, communicating with different organs and tissues to regulate processes such as metabolism, growth, reproduction, and stress response.

One of the key players in this hormonal symphony is the hypothalamus, a region of the brain that acts as a control center for many bodily functions. The hypothalamus releases hormones that stimulate or inhibit the production of hormones by the pituitary gland, which in turn regulates the secretion of hormones by other glands in the body.

For example, when the body experiences stress, the hypothalamus signals the pituitary gland to release adrenocorticotropic hormone (ACTH), which stimulates the adrenal glands to release cortisol, the body's primary stress hormone.[4] Cortisol triggers a cascade of physiological responses, including increased heart rate, elevated blood pressure, and heightened alertness, preparing the body to respond to the perceived threat.

Similarly, hormones play a crucial role in regulating mood and emotions. Serotonin, for example, is a neurotransmitter that helps regulate mood, sleep, and appetite. Imbalances in serotonin levels have been linked to mood disorders such as depression and anxiety.

When hormone levels fluctuate, whether due to natural hormonal cycles, stress, or medical conditions, it can have profound effects on the brain and overall well-being. For example, fluctuations in estrogen and progesterone levels during the menstrual cycle can affect mood, energy levels, and cognitive function in some women.

Similarly, imbalances in thyroid hormone levels can lead to symptoms such as fatigue, depression, and cognitive impairment. In conditions such as hypothyroidism, where thyroid hormone levels are low, individuals may experience symptoms such as sluggishness, weight gain, and depression. Conversely, in conditions such as hyperthyroidism, where thyroid hormone levels are elevated, individuals may experience symptoms such as anxiety, irritability, and insomnia.

In summary, the brain's interaction with hormones is a dynamic and tightly regulated process that plays a critical role in maintaining homeostasis and regulating a wide range of bodily functions.

When hormone levels are disrupted, whether due to natural fluctuations or underlying medical conditions, it can have profound effects on the brain and overall health.

The Dopamine

Dopamine is a neurotransmitter—a chemical messenger in the brain—that plays a key role in reward-motivated behavior, pleasure, and reinforcement learning.[5] It's often referred to as the "feel-good" hormone because it's released in response to pleasurable activities, such as eating delicious food, engaging in enjoyable activities, or experiencing social interactions.

In the context of addiction, including pornography addiction, dopamine's role becomes particularly significant. When a person engages in activities that they find pleasurable, such as viewing pornography, dopamine is released in the brain's reward pathway. This surge of dopamine creates a sensation of pleasure and reinforces the behavior, making the individual more likely to repeat it in the future.

However, with repeated exposure to highly stimulating activities, such as excessive pornography use, the brain's reward system can become dysregulated.[6] Over time, the brain may become desensitized to the effects of dopamine, requiring increasingly larger doses of stimulation to achieve the same level of pleasure. This phenomenon is known as tolerance.

Additionally, prolonged exposure to high levels of dopamine can lead to changes in the brain's structure and function, particularly in areas associated with motivation, reward, and impulse control. This can contribute to the development of addictive behaviors, as individuals become increasingly reliant on the addictive substance or activity to feel pleasure and avoid negative emotions.

The reconstruction of dopamine pathways in the brain is a crucial aspect of addiction recovery.

When individuals abstain from addictive behaviors, such as pornography use, their brain chemistry gradually begins to normalize. Dopamine receptors become more sensitive, and the brain's reward system becomes less reliant on external sources of stimulation.

However, rebuilding dopamine pathways takes time and effort. It often involves engaging in healthy, pleasurable activities that naturally boost dopamine levels, such as exercise, socializing, and pursuing hobbies and interests. Therapy and support groups can also be invaluable resources for individuals recovering from addiction, providing guidance, encouragement, and strategies for managing cravings and triggers.

By fostering a supportive environment and adopting healthy coping mechanisms, individuals can gradually rewire their brains and reclaim their lives from the grip of addiction. While the road to recovery may be challenging, the rewards—greater emotional well-being, improved relationships, and a renewed sense of purpose—are well worth the effort.

Testosterone

Testosterone is a hormone primarily produced in the testicles in males and in smaller amounts in the ovaries in females. It plays a crucial role in the development of male reproductive tissues, such as the testes and prostate, as well as promoting secondary sexual characteristics[7] like muscle mass, bone density, and body hair growth. In both males and females, testosterone also contributes to libido, mood regulation, and overall well-being.

In the context of pornography, there is ongoing debate and research regarding the effects of pornography consumption on testosterone levels. Some studies suggest that short-term exposure to sexual stimuli, such as viewing pornographic images or videos, may temporarily increase testosterone levels in both men and women. This transient rise in testosterone is believed to be part of the body's natural response to sexual arousal and may contribute to heightened sexual desire and arousal in the short term.

However, long-term or chronic exposure to pornography may have different effects on testosterone levels. Some research suggests that excessive pornography use may lead to desensitization of the brain's reward system, including the hypothalamic-pituitary-gonadal (HPG) axis, which regulates testosterone production.[8] This desensitization may result in a blunted response to sexual stimuli, leading to decreased sexual arousal and libido over time.

Additionally, pornography addiction and compulsive pornography use may contribute to psychological and emotional factors that can affect testosterone levels. Chronic stress, anxiety, and depression, which are common co-occurring conditions with pornography addiction, have been associated with disruptions in the HPG axis and decreased testosterone levels.

It's important to note that the relationship between pornography use and testosterone levels is complex and multifaceted, and more research is needed to fully understand the mechanisms involved. Additionally, individual responses to pornography may vary, and factors such as frequency of use, duration of exposure, and underlying psychological factors may influence the effects on testosterone levels.

Overall, while short-term exposure to pornography may temporarily increase testosterone levels as part of the body's natural response to sexual arousal, long-term or chronic exposure may have negative effects on testosterone production and sexual function. As with any behavior, moderation and mindful consumption are key to maintaining overall health and well-being.

The Terrifying Impact of Pornography Addiction on Psychological Health In the dark recesses of addiction lies a horror that few dare to confront: the insidious grip of pornography and its devastating effects on psychological health. As we delve into the depths of this nightmare, we are forced to confront a chilling hypothesis: that an individual, ensnared by the siren song of pornography, is doomed to suffer a fate worse than death.

Imagine, if you will, a person consumed by an addiction so powerful, so all-encompassing, that it robs them of their very humanity. Their once-vibrant libido, now a mere shadow of its former self, lies dormant, suffocated by the relentless onslaught of explicit imagery and hypersexualized fantasies.

As the addiction tightens its grip, the individual finds themselves trapped in a nightmarish cycle of despair and degradation. Their relationships crumble beneath the weight of their addiction, as intimacy and connection are replaced by emptiness and shame. Their ability to experience pleasure, once a source of joy and fulfillment, now lies shattered and broken, a casualty of their relentless pursuit of carnal gratification.

But the horror does not end there. As the addiction festers and grows, so too do the desires of the afflicted. No longer satisfied with conventional forms of sexual expression, they find themselves drawn to ever more depraved and taboo acts. Group sex, homosexual encounters, even relationships with inanimate objects—nothing is off-limits in their desperate quest for stimulation.

And so, the descent into madness continues, as the individual is consumed by a maelstrom of desire and despair. Their once-normal desires twisted and perverted by the relentless onslaught of pornography, they become lost souls adrift in a sea of depravity and dysfunction.

But perhaps the most terrifying aspect of all is the realization that this nightmare could happen to anyone. In a world where pornography is just a click away, no one is immune to its seductive allure. It preys upon the vulnerable, the lonely, the lost, ensnaring them in its web of deception and despair.

As we confront the chilling reality of pornography addiction, let us not shy away from the terror that lurks within. Let us sound the alarm, raise our voices in protest, and shine a light into the darkest corners of addiction. For only by confronting the horror head-on can we hope to break free from its suffocating grasp and reclaim our humanity once more.

Feelings of addiction

1. Loneliness: Porn addicts often experience profound feelings of loneliness, despite being surrounded by others. Their addiction isolates them, creating a barrier between themselves and their loved ones. They may struggle to form genuine connections with others, leading to a sense of alienation and social withdrawal.
2. Feeling Sad: Porn addiction can contribute to feelings of sadness and despair. As the addiction progresses, individuals

may find themselves caught in a cycle of shame and guilt, perpetuated by their inability to control their behavior. This sense of hopelessness can weigh heavily on their emotional well-being, leading to persistent feelings of sadness and melancholy.

3. Feeling of Lack of Self-Confidence: Porn addiction can erode self-confidence and self-esteem. As individuals become increasingly reliant on pornography for sexual gratification, they may develop unrealistic expectations of themselves and their partners. This can lead to feelings of inadequacy and self-doubt, undermining their confidence in both their appearance and their abilities.

4. Feeling Depressed: Chronic pornography use has been associated with an increased risk of depression. The dopamine surges triggered by pornographic stimuli can create a temporary sense of euphoria, followed by a crash as dopamine levels plummet. Over time, this cycle can contribute to dysregulation of the brain's reward system, leading to persistent feelings of depression and dysphoria.

5. Feeling Unable to Cope with a Partner Sexually and Emotionally: Porn addiction can strain intimate relationships, making it difficult for individuals to connect with their partners sexually and emotionally. They may struggle to maintain arousal and intimacy with a real-life partner, preferring the artificial stimulation provided by pornography. This can lead to feelings of frustration, resentment, and ultimately, the breakdown of the relationship.

6. Feeling Tired: Excessive pornography use can disrupt sleep patterns and contribute to feelings of fatigue and exhaustion. Individuals may find themselves staying up late to indulge in their addiction, sacrificing valuable rest and recovery time. This can take a toll on their physical and mental well-being, leaving them feeling constantly tired and rundown.

7. Bad Memory and Distraction: Porn addiction can impair cognitive function, leading to difficulties with concentration,

memory, and focus. Individuals may find themselves easily distracted and forgetful, struggling to retain information and stay organized. This cognitive fog can further exacerbate feelings of frustration and inadequacy, perpetuating the cycle of addiction.

Overall, the feelings experienced by porn addicts are varied and complex, reflecting the profound impact of addiction on their emotional, psychological, and interpersonal well-being. Addressing these feelings requires a holistic approach that encompasses therapy, support, and a commitment to recovery.

CHAPTER 4:
THE DEVIL

Victims of Pornography - From Young to Old, Women to Men

In the sinister world of pornography, there are no boundaries, no limits to the harm it can inflict. From the innocence of youth to the wisdom of old age, no one is immune to its insidious allure. Men and women, young and old alike, find themselves ensnared in its web of exploitation and degradation.

At its core, pornography is a form of exploitation, preying upon the vulnerabilities and insecurities of its victims. For young people, still navigating the complexities of adolescence, pornography can distort their perceptions of sex and relationships, setting unrealistic expectations and fostering unhealthy attitudes towards intimacy.[1]

But the harm doesn't end there. Women, too, are targeted by the porn industry, objectified and dehumanized for the pleasure of others. From mainstream pornography to the darkest corners of the internet, women are reduced to mere objects of desire, stripped of their humanity and dignity.[2] And let us not forget the men who fall victim to pornography's siren song. Trapped in a cycle of addiction and shame, they find themselves powerless to resist its allure, their relationships and self-worth crumbling beneath the weight of their obsession.[3]

But perhaps the most tragic victims of all are the elderly, whose vulnerability is exploited for profit by an industry devoid of conscience.

Pornography, with its promise of excitement and arousal, becomes yet another weapon in the arsenal of those who seek to prey upon the vulnerable and powerless.[4]

In the face of such rampant exploitation, it is easy to feel hopeless and overwhelmed. But we must not despair. By shining a light into the darkness, by speaking out against injustice and exploitation, we can empower ourselves and others to break free from the chains of pornography and reclaim our dignity and humanity

Lily!

In the heart of a bustling city, amidst the neon lights and throngs of people, lived Lily, a young woman with dreams as big as the skyscrapers that towered above her. From the outside, she seemed to have it all—a promising career, a loving family, and a circle of friends who adored her. But beneath her confident exterior lurked a dark secret, a secret that threatened to unravel her carefully constructed facade.

It started innocently enough, a casual click on a website late one night when boredom and curiosity got the best of her. What began as a fleeting moment of excitement soon spiraled into an all-consuming obsession, as Lily found herself drawn deeper and deeper into the world of pornography.

At first, it was just a harmless escape from the stresses of everyday life, a way to unwind and indulge in a guilty pleasure. But as the addiction took hold, it began to consume every waking moment, leaving Lily feeling empty and ashamed. She tried to quit, to break free from the grip of pornography, but each attempt only left her feeling more powerless and defeated.

As her addiction worsened, Lily's life began to unravel. She became withdrawn and distant, retreating into a world of fantasy and illusion where the only thing that mattered was the next hit of dopamine. Her relationships suffered, as friends and family grew increasingly concerned about her well-being. She pushed them away, unable to face the shame and guilt that consumed her.

But even as she spiraled deeper into despair, a glimmer of hope remained. Through the darkness, Lily found the courage to seek help, to confront her addiction head-on and reclaim her life from its suffocating grasp. With the support of loved ones and the guidance of therapists and support groups, she embarked on a journey of recovery, determined to break free from the chains of addiction and reclaim her dignity and humanity.

It was a long and difficult road, filled with setbacks and struggles, but with each passing day, Lily grew stronger and more resilient. She learned to confront her demons, to face her fears and insecurities head-on, and in doing so, she discovered a strength within herself that she never knew existed.

In the end, Lily emerged victorious, a survivor of the darkest depths of addiction. Though the scars of her past remained, she refused to let them define her, choosing instead to embrace the future with hope and optimism. And as she looked out at the world with eyes that were clear and unclouded by shame, she knew that she was finally free.[5]

The Impact

The impact of pornography spans across different demographics and societies, affecting individuals in various ways. Women often face the brunt of unrealistic portrayals in pornography, leading to feelings of inadequacy, low self-esteem, and body dissatisfaction. Mothers may find their relationships strained as pornography addiction can overshadow familial responsibilities, creating a toxic environment for children.[6]

For wives, trust and intimacy in marriages can be eroded by a partner's addiction, fostering insecurity and resentment. Similarly, fathers may struggle with shame and secrecy, isolating themselves from loved ones.

Men, despite being primary consumers, aren't immune to pornography's effects. Addiction can lead to erectile dysfunction, reduced libido, and difficulty forming genuine connections. Students may experience academic and social repercussions, including impaired cognitive function and social isolation.[7]

On a societal level, pornography contributes to shaping attitudes towards sex, relationships, and gender roles. Its widespread availability normalizes violence and exploitation, straining healthcare systems, social services, and law enforcement agencies.[8]

Overall, addressing pornography's harms requires a multifaceted approach encompassing education, prevention, treatment, and support for affected individuals and communities.

The industry

The pornography industry, often referred to as the adult entertainment industry, is a vast and lucrative business that encompasses a wide range of media, including videos, magazines, websites, live performances, and more. While it's difficult to obtain precise financial data due to the secretive nature of the industry and its often unregulated status, estimates suggest that it generates billions of dollars in revenue annually.

1. Revenue Streams: The pornography industry generates revenue through various channels, including subscription-based websites, pay-per-view content, advertising, merchandise sales, live performances, and licensing agreements. Additionally, the rise of streaming services and online platforms has expanded the industry's reach and profitability.
2. Global Reach: The pornography industry is a global phenomenon, with production and consumption occurring in countries around the world. While the United States has traditionally been a major player in the industry, other countries, including Brazil, Japan, and the Netherlands, also have significant adult entertainment markets.[9]

3. Internet Proliferation: The advent of the internet revolutionized the pornography industry, making it more accessible and widespread than ever before. With the click of a button, consumers can access a vast array of pornographic content from the comfort of their own homes, bypassing traditional distribution channels and regulations.

4. Tech and Innovation: The pornography industry has embraced technological innovation, leveraging advances in video streaming, virtual reality, and interactive content to enhance the consumer experience. From immersive virtual reality experiences to live webcam shows, the industry is constantly evolving to meet the demands of its audience.[10]

5. Controversy and Ethics: Despite its profitability, the pornography industry is not without controversy. Critics raise concerns about exploitation, objectification, and the impact of pornography on society, particularly its potential effects on attitudes towards sex, relationships, and gender roles. Additionally, the industry has faced scrutiny over issues such as piracy, child exploitation, and labor rights.

6. Economic Impact: While the pornography industry generates significant revenue for producers, performers, and distributors, its economic impact extends beyond direct financial gains. Pornography production stimulates demand for various goods and services, including equipment, talent, and marketing, contributing to economic activity in related industries.

7. Regulation and Legal Status: The pornography industry operates within a complex legal and regulatory framework, with laws varying widely from country to country. While some countries have strict regulations governing pornography production and distribution, others have more lenient or permissive policies. This patchwork of regulations can create challenges for producers and consumers alike, particularly in the age of online content sharing and global distribution.

The art and artists of the porn industry

The Jewish Influence in the Pornography Industry: Unveiling the pioneers I wish to clarify an important matter: I hold the Jewish religion in high regard as one of the Abrahamic faiths. We share a Semitic heritage, with roots in the Middle East, which is also the cradle of my own ancestry. The Jewish community, however, comprises two distinct groups with significant differences between them.

The first group consists of Jews who believe in God, respect others, and perform good deeds. I see no distinction between them and my own family and friends; I consider them as fellow adherents of divine religions with whom I share many values.

On the other hand, there is Zionism, a movement marked by a lack of compassion and morality, driven by unrestrained greed and avarice. This faction has entangled itself in the pornography industry and engages in conspiracies that harm Jews, Christians, Muslims, and all believers in God. Their goal is to undermine virtue and promote vice.

In this article, I will delve into how Zionists have exerted control over the pornography industry and discuss the European Jews who have adopted Judaism in various forms. It is important to note that I do not generalize this to all Jews, as goodness exists everywhere. However, those with a discerning heart and common sense will recognize a Zionist by their actions and malevolence.

In this book, when I refer to Jews involved in corrupting the youth and scattering their minds, I am specifically addressing Zionists, not the beloved Jewish believers who uphold their faith with integrity.

The pornography industry has long been a subject of intrigue and controversy, with its origins and evolution intertwined with the contributions of numerous individuals. Among these figures, the influence of the Jewish community stands out prominently, as men and women of Jewish-Zionist descent played significant roles in shaping the landscape of adult entertainment.[11]

From the post-war era onwards, the rise of pornographic magazines and outlets saw a surge in Jewish-Zionist involvement, with names like Robin Sturman emerging as key figures in the industry.

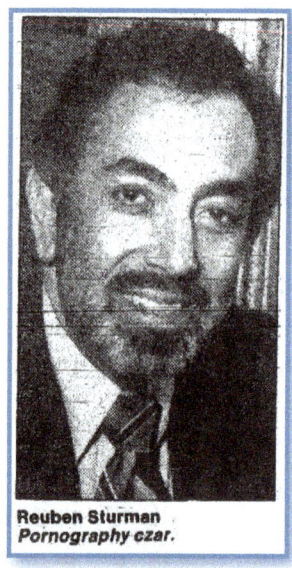

Reuben Sturman
Pornography czar.

Sturman, often hailed as the "Walt Disney of pornography," wielded immense influence as a producer, controlling a vast empire that dominated much of the pornographic production in the

United States during the 1970s. His Orthodox Jewish background added to the intrigue, as he became known as the patriarch of the global porn industry, symbolizing the intersection of religion and commerce in the adult entertainment world.

But Sturman was not alone in his influence. Throughout history, men and women of Jewish-Zionist descent have made significant contributions to the pornography industry, both behind the scenes and in front of the camera. From directors and producers to performers and entrepreneurs, individuals of Jewish heritage have played pivotal roles in shaping the content, distribution, and consumption of adult entertainment.

The reasons for the disproportionate representation of Jewish individuals in the pornography industry are complex and multifaceted. Some attribute it to cultural factors, including a tradition of entrepreneurship and a willingness to challenge societal norms. Others point to historical factors, such as the marginalization of Jewish communities in mainstream industries, leading them to seek opportunities in alternative sectors like adult entertainment.

Regardless of the reasons, the Jewish influence in the pornography industry is undeniable, with men and women of Jewish-Zionist descent leaving an indelible mark on the world of adult entertainment.

While their contributions have often been met with controversy and scrutiny, they have also reshaped the industry and challenged prevailing attitudes towards sexuality, identity, and freedom of expression.

As we continue to explore the complex dynamics of the pornography industry, it is essential to recognize the diverse array of individuals who have contributed to its evolution. By acknowledging the role of Jewish-Zionist pioneers in shaping the landscape of adult entertainment.

European Jews and the industry

("If you're welcomed into the porn industry, it's unbelievable. It's an extended family... There are way too many Jews involved in it!"

(A group of actors and actresses in the porn industry, in their meeting with American psychologist Robert Stoller)

In 2016, the Israeli Knesset passed a bill requiring Internet Service Providers (ISPs) to block pornographic websites throughout the country due to the "harm they cause to children and society, especially as accessing pornographic sites now is easier than buying ice cream at the local market. This compelled the Jewish-Zionist state to act to protect minors from this danger."

This law raised a valid question because of its strange paradox: how do Jews block pornography in their country while being the pioneers who inflated the pornographic industry and invested in it from the beginning? Some people attempted to present historical facts about the role of Jews in the pornographic industry, but most of them were either attacked for anti-Semitism and inciting violence or faced censorship by having their videos deleted from the internet and YouTube.

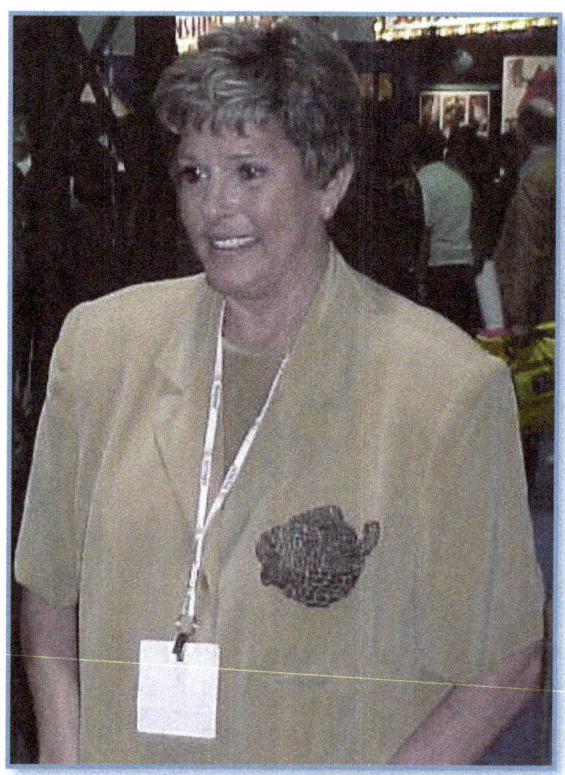

Gloria Leonard - wikidata.org

Early Investments

When the pornographic industry began to intensify in the early 20th century, it wasn't as it is now. With the possibility of accessing pornographic websites at any moment today, internet and video technologies were not available in the early 20th century. Therefore, the industry relied on other outlets to promote pornography, most of which are now obsolete but still exist to some extent, such as phone sex lines, erotic magazines, adult theaters, and pornographic videotapes. Jews dominated most, if not all, of these areas. According to Time magazine, Gloria Leonard, the inventor of phone sex lines, was Zionist. Throughout her pornographic career, Leonard always identified herself as: "a nice Jewish girl from the neighborhoods of New York." The story of phone sex calls began when Leonard decided in 1977 to invest her fame in the pornographic industry as an actress and as the editor-in-chief of "High Society" pornographic magazine to promote this new genre of pornography, and the demand for this new genre exceeded imagination.

Leonard was not unique as a Zionist editor-in-chief of a pornographic magazine, but this was prevalent at that time. Even the famous magazine "Playboy," founded in the mid-1950s, had a strong Jewish presence in its editorial team from its inception. To the extent that one of its Zionist editors, Nat Lehrman, recalls, saying: "The entire team, practically speaking, was Zionist. We were the dominant ones, perhaps the brightest!"

After the spread of pornographic magazines and outlets for sale in the post-war period from 1950 onwards, Jewish influence in the industry increased. The name Rubin Sturman emerged and became the most famous producer in the United States, earning him the nickname "the Walt Disney of the pornographic industry." Throughout the entire 1970s, Sturman owned a massive empire that controlled most of the pornographic production circulating in the entire United States, to the extent that - alone - he owned more than 200 pornographic magazine stores.

According to Nathan Abrams, an American history professor at Aberdeen University: "No one could get pornographic content without passing through Sturman."

Sturman was a traditional Jew and was considered the spiritual father of the entire global pornographic industry. He once stated to one of his interviewers: "If you want to know how the pornographic industry started, you're looking at the person who started it!" Despite Sturman's immense wealth, with some estimates suggesting he earned a million dollars a day, his greed knew no bounds. In his later years, he was charged with embezzlement and tax evasion and was sentenced to prison until he died in 1997.

Technological Advancement and Persistent Domination As technology has advanced, attention has shifted from images to videos due to the affordability of cameras, prompting Jews to capitalize on this opportunity to transition from still imagery to motion pictures. Pornography penetrated video tapes and gained significant popularity. Mike Kulish, a Jewish pornographic director, asserts that Jews were the first to introduce popular video technology to the industry, stating, "Jews made radical changes in the pornography industry, founding companies that produced DVDs, VHS tapes, and Betamax, revolutionizing the promotion of pornography among nations."

He continues: "Simply put, all pioneers in the pornography business are mostly Zionist, have Zionist connections, or at times worked under Zionist... Zionist have dominated the industry, or in other words, all companies had to go through Zionist."

Thus, Zionist dominance in the pornography industry peaked in the seventies and eighties. Zionist not only controlled production but also expanded into pornographic representation. It is widely known that most male pornographic actors in the seventies and eighties were Jewish- Zionist. Among these actors, one of the most famous, if not the most famous, was the American

Jew Ron Jeremy, dubbed the "legend of the pornographic industry," as he holds the Guinness World Record for the most appearances in pornographic films, appearing in over 2000 films alone.

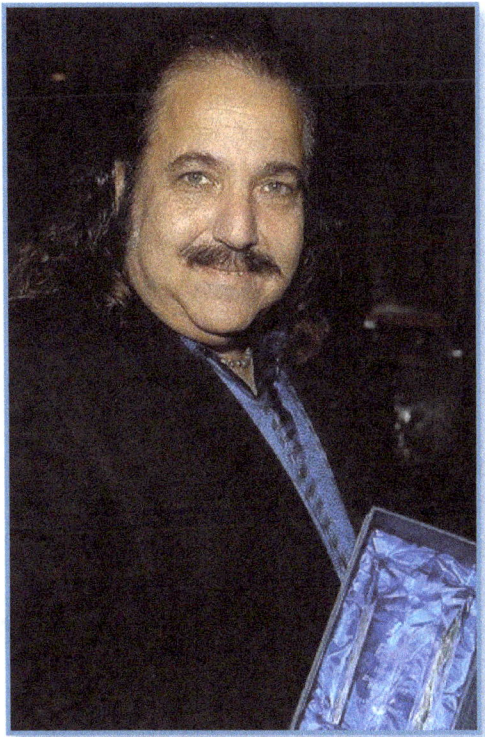

Ron Jeremy - wikipedia.org

Domination Continues

In the early nineties, the promise of the internet revolution emerged. One young producer, Seth Warshawsky, established Internet Entertainment Group (IEG) to market pornography through live broadcasts and recorded videos. The company started with modest offerings but quickly expanded to become the largest pornography company on the internet by 1998, with annual profits reaching $50 million.

As a result of this pornographic empire's expansion, Warshawsky became the symbol of internet pornography in all media. According to William Pierce, an American physics professor, Warshawsky was dubbed "the Bill Gates of online pornography" because he owned many major pornographic websites.

On the other hand, during the nineties, the activities of the Adult Video News (AVN) network covering the pornography industry expanded. This network, founded by Paul Fishbein in the mid-eighties, has become the premier network in its field, hosting events, presenting awards to producers and actors akin to the Oscars, holding competitions, and publishing news and advertisements related to the pornography industry.

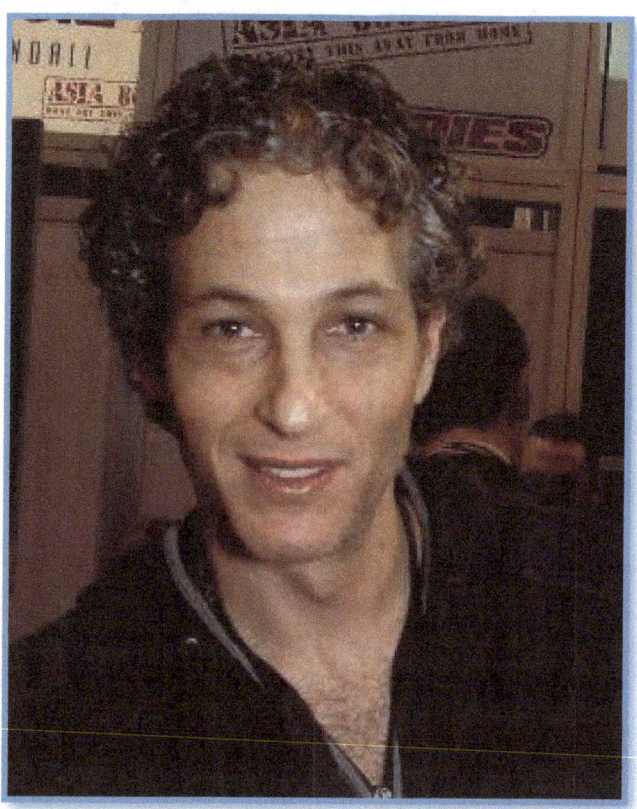

Seymour Butts - wikipedia.org

Between AVN and IEG, a new color of pornography emerged in 1991, which would become the most famous color these days. The story begins when Jewish businessman Seymour Butts went to a nude club and hired a dancer, borrowed a video camera for 24 hours, and filmed a pornographic clip with the dancer. The clip was poor quality and received almost no success.

However, over time, Butts managed to strike deals with several companies, and within a few years, he became the "king of violent pornography." This type of pornography is characterized by extreme violence and repulsive tastes. Butts currently owns a pornographic empire, with his films generating profits at least ten times their production cost.

In the context of discussing pornographic economic empires, many analysts consider the contemporary revival of the Sturman empire to be the 57-year-old Jewish man Steven Hirsch, known as the "Donald Trump of the pornographic industry" and the CEO of Vivid Entertainment, dubbed "Microsoft of pornography." Forbes magazine reported that Vivid "Controls 30% of the pornographic market in the United States." Surprisingly, the largest competitor to Vivid Entertainment is Wicked Pictures, run by Steve Orenstein, who is also Jewish, competing with Steven Hirsch.

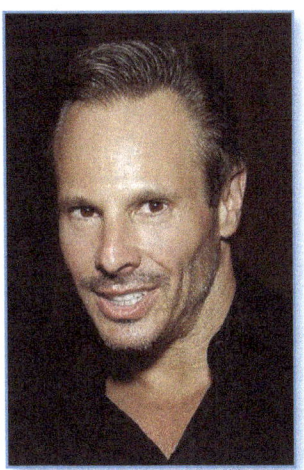

Steven Hirsch - wikipedia.org

Reasons for Jewish Infiltration in the Pornography Industry

Entering the industry may seem acceptable within the framework of free market mechanisms. Still, the problem lies in the disproportionate domination of this industry, not at all commensurate with their population in the American state. According to American Jew Luke Ford, "Although Jews make up only 2% of the American population, they control the pornography industry."

The question remains: What drove Jews to this sacred invasion of the pornography industry? In 2000, the Jerusalem Post newspaper reported that "most publishers and itinerant booksellers of so-called erotic and pornographic literature were Jewish, and most of these Jews were Germans who learned printing in the old country." With the migration of Jews from Europe to the United States in the early twentieth century, Jews entered the pornography industry "as individuals seeking to achieve the American dream," as American lawyer Abraham Foxman put it. Nathan Abrams, a professor of American history at the University of Aberdeen in Britain and a religious Jew, says: "Jews entered the pornography industry because at the beginning of the twentieth century, one did not need a lot of money to start a pornography business."

Is there a deeper reason than just financial profit and cheap production costs? Researchers list reasons such as rebellion against conservative values, a desire to corrupt people, and extreme Google Image (Al Goldstein) openness from European concentration camp to American freedom. However, no one was more outspoken than Jewish pornographic producer AL Goldstein. When asked why Jews dominated the pornography industry, his response was very clear: "The only reason Jews participate in the porn industry is because we hate Jesus Christ... Porn then became a means of desecrating Christian culture because it quickly penetrates American homes."

Of course, Goldstein's view cannot be generalized to all porn producers, but it appears to be a remarkably widespread and recurring view in the porn medium, as Luke Ford writes: "In the early twentieth century, Jews became involved in pornography out of reactionary hatred of Christians. They attempted to subvert mainstream American values in At that time, it seems that they actually succeeded in doing... Pornographic films now are not related to what is aesthetic and romantic, but rather to what is shocking to the viewer."

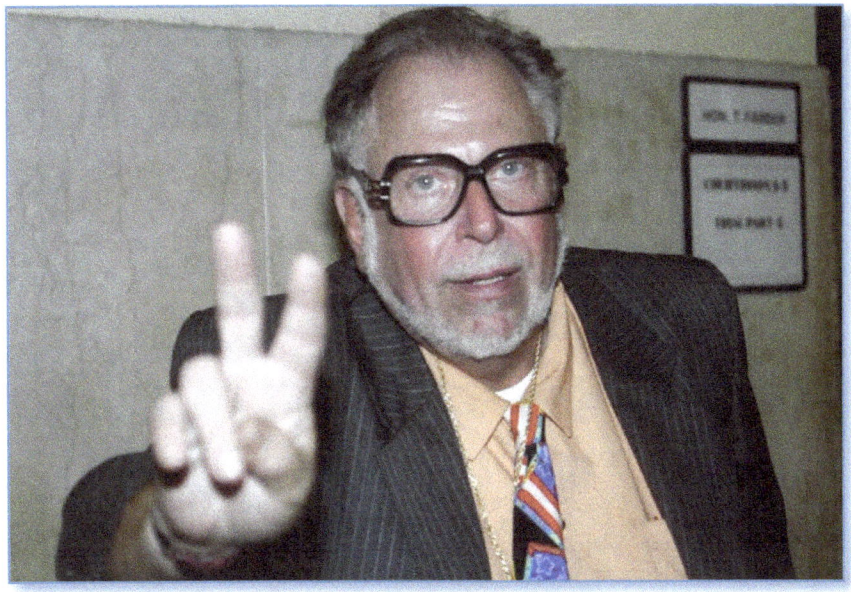

Google Image (Al Goldstein)

In every aspect of the pornographic industry, it began with the control of pornographic stores, followed by the invention of sexual conversations, then the integration of videotapes into the industry, and after that the Internet revolution ignited and the introduction of live-broadcast pornography ended with the Jews sitting on the throne of pornographic economic empires. We may not be able to control Jewish dominance of the industry, but what we can control is simply our viewing and consumption of their products.)[12]

CHAPTER 5:
"YES, I CAN QUIT."

Free will

Human free will refers to the capacity of individuals to make choices and decisions without being determined by external factors or forces.[1] It is the ability to act independently and to choose one's own course of action based on personal values, beliefs, and desires. Free will implies that individuals have control over their actions and can exercise autonomy in shaping their lives.

When it comes to addiction to pornography, free will plays a significant role. Addiction is often characterized by compulsive behavior despite negative consequences. In the case of pornography addiction, individuals may feel a lack of control over their consumption, leading to excessive and harmful use of pornography.

However, free will is not completely overridden by addiction. While addiction can impair decision-making processes and make it challenging to resist urges, individuals still retain some degree of agency and can exert control over their actions. Overcoming addiction to pornography requires harnessing this free will to initiate and sustain change.[2]

Here are some steps that individuals struggling with pornography addiction can take to overcome this challenge:

1. Self-awareness: Recognize and acknowledge that there is a problem. Reflect on how pornography use is impacting various aspects of your life, including relationships, mental health, and overall well-being.

   Self-awareness is a crucial component in the recovery from porn addiction. It involves recognizing and understanding one's thoughts, emotions, and behaviors related to pornography use.[3] By becoming more self-aware, individuals can identify the underlying causes and triggers of their addiction, which is essential for effective recovery.[4] Here's how self-awareness can contribute to overcoming porn addiction:

a. Identifying Triggers:

- Self-awareness helps individuals recognize the specific situations, emotions, or thoughts that trigger the urge to consume pornography. Understanding these triggers allows for the development of strategies to avoid or cope with them in healthier ways.

b. Understanding the Impact:

- By being self-aware, individuals can see the negative consequences of their addiction on various aspects of their lives, such as relationships, work, mental health, and overall well-being. This awareness can motivate them to seek change and commit to recovery.

c. Recognizing Patterns:

- Self-awareness enables individuals to observe patterns in their behavior, such as the times of day or emotional states when they are most likely to use pornography. Recognizing these patterns can help in creating a plan to interrupt and change these habits.

d. Increasing Emotional Intelligence:

- Developing self-awareness enhances emotional intelligence, allowing individuals to better understand and manage their emotions. This can reduce the reliance on pornography as a coping mechanism for dealing with stress, loneliness, or other negative emotions.

e. Fostering Accountability:

- Being self-aware encourages personal accountability. Individuals who are aware of their actions and their consequences are more likely to take responsibility for their recovery and make conscious efforts to change.

f. Enhancing Self-Control:

- Self-awareness helps in developing self-control. By being mindful of their thoughts and urges, individuals can practice delaying gratification and making more deliberate choices rather than acting on impulse.

g. Setting Realistic Goals:

- A self-aware individual can set realistic and attainable goals for reducing or eliminating pornography use. They can monitor their progress, celebrate small victories, and adjust their strategies as needed.

h. Improving Self-Compassion:

- Self-awareness includes recognizing one's flaws and struggles without excessive self- criticism. This fosters self-compassion, which is important for maintaining motivation and resilience during the recovery process.

i. Seeking Support:

- Self-aware individuals are more likely to recognize when they need help and seek support from friends, family, or professionals. They understand that recovery is not a solitary journey and that external support can provide valuable insights and encouragement.

j. Building a Stronger Sense of Identity:

- Through self-awareness, individuals can explore their values, beliefs, and goals beyond pornography. This helps in building a stronger sense of identity and purpose, reducing the reliance on pornography for fulfillment or escape.

Practical Steps to Enhance Self-Awareness:

- Mindfulness Meditation: Regular practice of mindfulness can help individuals become more aware of their thoughts and feelings without judgment.
- Journaling: Writing down thoughts, emotions, and behaviors related to pornography use can provide insights into patterns and triggers.
- Therapy: Working with a therapist can help individuals explore underlying issues contributing to addiction and develop self-awareness.
- Reflection: Regular self-reflection, such as taking time each day to review actions and emotions, can increase self-awareness.

2. Seek support: Reach out to trusted friends, family members, or professionals for support. Joining a support group or seeking therapy can provide valuable guidance and encouragement in overcoming addiction.

Seeking and receiving help is highly effective for individuals struggling with porn addiction. The process of reaching out for support and accepting assistance can provide crucial resources, guidance, and encouragement[5] that are often necessary for overcoming addiction. Here's how seeking and receiving help can be effective:

a. Professional Therapy and Counseling:

- Expert Guidance: Professional therapists and counselors who specialize in addiction can provide evidence-based treatment methods, such as Cognitive Behavioral Therapy (CBT), which helps individuals change their thinking patterns and behaviors related to pornography use.[6]
- Identifying Root Causes: Therapists can help individuals uncover underlying issues, such as trauma, anxiety, or depression, that may be contributing to their addiction.
- Developing Coping Strategies: Professionals can teach effective coping mechanisms to manage triggers and stressors without resorting to pornography.

b. Support Groups:

- Shared Experiences: Support groups like Sex Addicts Anonymous (SAA) or Porn Addicts Anonymous (PAA) offer a safe space where individuals can share their experiences and challenges with others who understand their struggles.
- Accountability: Regular meetings and check-ins with group members can provide accountability, which is critical for maintaining progress and preventing relapse.
- Emotional Support: Being part of a support group reduces feelings of isolation and provides emotional support, which can be comforting and motivating.

c. Educational Resources:

- Increased Awareness: Books, articles, and online resources about porn addiction can help individuals understand the nature of their addiction and the impact it has on their brain and behavior.

- Practical Tools: Educational resources often include practical tools and exercises for managing cravings and building healthier habits.

d. Family and Friends:

- Emotional Support: Loved ones can offer emotional support, understanding, and encouragement, which can boost an individual's confidence and motivation to recover.
- Accountability Partners: Friends and family can act as accountability partners, helping the individual stay on track with their recovery goals.
- Creating a Supportive Environment: A supportive home environment, free from triggers and stressors, can significantly aid the recovery process.

e. Medical Assistance:

- Medication: In some cases, medication may be prescribed to help manage underlying mental health issues such as depression or anxiety, which can contribute to porn addiction.
- Medical Advice: Healthcare providers can offer advice on maintaining overall well- being, which is crucial for recovery.

f. Spiritual Guidance:

- Moral Support: For some individuals, spiritual leaders or faith-based counseling can provide moral support and a sense of purpose in their recovery journey.
- Community Support: Faith communities often offer a network of support and accountability.

g. Online Forums and Apps:

- Anonymity: Online forums and apps offer a degree of anonymity that might make it easier for individuals to seek help.
- 24/7 Availability: Many online resources are available 24/7, providing immediate support when needed.

HCustomized Recovery Plans:

- Personalized Treatment: Receiving help allows for the development of a personalized recovery plan that addresses the specific needs and circumstances of the individual.
- Progress Monitoring: Regular check-ins with professionals can help track progress and make necessary adjustments to the recovery plan.

Benefits of Seeking and Receiving Help:

- Breaking the Cycle of Isolation: Addiction often leads to isolation. Seeking help breaks this cycle and connects individuals with supportive communities.
- Empowerment and Motivation: Support from others can empower individuals to take control of their recovery and stay motivated.
- Building Resilience: Through therapy and support, individuals can build resilience and develop skills to handle life's challenges without resorting to pornography.
- Preventing Relapse: Ongoing support and accountability are crucial in preventing relapse and maintaining long-term sobriety.

Overcoming Barriers to Seeking Help:

- Reducing Stigma: Education about porn addiction can help reduce the stigma and encourage more people to seek help.
- Promoting Awareness: Raising awareness about the availability and effectiveness of support options can motivate individuals to take the first step towards recovery.

3. Set goals: Establish clear and achievable goals for reducing or eliminating pornography use. Break down goals into smaller steps and celebrate progress along the way.

Setting goals for recovery is a crucial strategy for porn addicts aiming to overcome their addiction. Establishing cl and track their progress effectively ear, achievable goals provides direction, motivation, and a sense of purpose[7], making the recovery process more structured and manageable. Here's how porn addicts can set effective goals for recovery and the benefits associated with this practice:

Steps to Setting Goals for Recovery

1. Identify Long-Term Objectives:

- Vision of Success: Define what successful recovery looks like. This could include complete abstinence from pornography, improved relationships, or enhanced self-esteem.
- Personal Motivation: Understand personal reasons for wanting to recover, such as restoring trust in relationships, improving mental health, or achieving professional goals.

2. Break Down into Short-Term Goals:

- Manageable Steps: Break the long-term objective into smaller, more manageable short- term goals. This could be

daily or weekly targets, such as reducing the frequency of porn consumption or engaging in alternative activities.
- Incremental Progress: Focus on gradual progress to avoid feeling overwhelmed. Celebrate small victories to stay motivated.

3. Set SMART Goals:

- Specific: Clearly define the goal. Instead of saying "reduce porn usage," specify "limit porn viewing to once a week."
- Measurable: Ensure the goal can be quantified. This helps in tracking progress and staying accountable.
- Achievable: Set realistic goals that are attainable given the current circumstances.
- Relevant: Ensure the goals are meaningful and directly contribute to the overall recovery.
- Time-Bound: Establish a timeline for achieving the goals. For example, "reduce porn viewing by 50% within the next month."

4. Develop an Action Plan:

- Concrete Steps: Outline specific actions required to achieve each goal. This might include attending support group meetings, practicing mindfulness, or seeking therapy.
- Resources and Support: Identify the resources needed, such as support groups, counseling, or educational materials.

5. Monitor and Adjust Goals:

- Regular Review: Periodically review progress towards goals. This helps in recognizing achievements and identifying areas needing adjustment.

- Flexibility: Be willing to adjust goals based on progress and changing circumstances. Recovery is not always linear, and adjustments are a part of the process.

Benefits of Setting Goals for Recovery

1. Provides Direction and Focus:

    - Clear Path: Goals provide a clear roadmap, helping addicts understand what steps to take next.
    - Avoiding Distractions: By focusing on specific objectives, individuals are less likely to get sidetracked.

2. Enhances Motivation:

    - Sense of Purpose: Goals give a sense of purpose and direction, which can enhance motivation.
    - Visible Progress: Tracking progress towards goals provides tangible evidence of improvement, boosting morale and determination.

3. Increases Accountability:

    - Self-Accountability: Setting goals creates a personal commitment to achieving them, increasing self-accountability.
    - External Accountability: Sharing goals with a therapist, support group, or trusted individuals can provide external accountability and encouragement.

4. Reduces Overwhelm:

    - Small Steps: Breaking recovery into smaller, achievable steps makes the process less overwhelming.
    - Manageable Tasks: Focusing on one goal at a time prevents the feeling of being burdened by the entirety of the recovery process.

5. Improves Self-Esteem:

    - Achieving Goals: Accomplishing set goals, even small ones, can significantly boost self- esteem and confidence.
    - Empowerment: Setting and achieving goals empowers addicts, reinforcing the belief that they can overcome their addiction.

6. Facilitates Positive Behavior Change:

    - Healthy Habits: Goals can encourage the development of healthy habits and coping mechanisms, such as exercise, hobbies, or social activities.
    - Replacement Activities: Identifying alternative activities to replace porn consumption can lead to a healthier, more balanced lifestyle.

7. Encourages Continuous Improvement:

    - Ongoing Growth: Regularly setting and achieving goals fosters a mindset of continuous improvement and personal growth.
    - Adapting to Change: As recovery progresses, goals can be adjusted to reflect new challenges and achievements, ensuring continuous forward movement.

Examples of Recovery Goals

- Daily Journaling: Write in a journal every day to reflect on triggers and emotions.
- Therapy Sessions: Attend therapy sessions once a week for the next three months.
- Support Group Participation: Participate in a support group meeting twice a week.
- Mindfulness Practice: Practice mindfulness or meditation for 15 minutes every day.

- Physical Activity: Engage in physical exercise three times a week to manage stress and improve mood.

In conclusion, setting goals for recovery from porn addiction is an effective strategy that provides structure, motivation, and a clear path forward. It helps addicts focus on actionable steps, track their progress, and build confidence through achievable milestones, ultimately leading to a successful recovery journey.

1. Develop coping strategies: Identify healthier ways to cope with stress, boredom, or negative emotions that may trigger the urge to consume pornography. This could include engaging in hobbies, exercise, mindfulness practices, or spending time with loved ones.
2. Create barriers: Take practical steps to limit access to pornography, such as using content filters or blocking software on devices, avoiding triggers, and setting boundaries around internet usage.
3. Replace negative habits with positive ones: Replace the time and energy spent on pornography with activities that promote personal growth, fulfillment, and connection with others.

Creating new habits to replace the bad habit of porn consumption is an essential strategy for reducing addiction. This involves identifying triggers, choosing healthier alternatives, and consistently practicing these new behaviors until they become ingrained.[9] Here's a detailed guide on how porn addicts can create and maintain new habits to reduce addiction:

Steps to Creating New Habits

1. Identify Triggers and Understand Patterns:

    - Awareness: Keep a journal to track when and why you feel the urge to watch porn. Note emotional states, specific times of day, and particular situations that act as triggers.

- Patterns: Identify recurring themes or patterns in your behavior that lead to porn consumption.

2. Choose Healthy Alternatives:

    - Activities: Select activities that you enjoy and can turn to when you feel the urge. These could include exercise, reading, hobbies, or spending time with friends.
    - Coping Mechanisms: Develop coping mechanisms for managing stress, boredom, loneliness, or other emotions that trigger porn use. This might involve practicing mindfulness, meditation, or engaging in creative outlets.

3. Set Specific, Achievable Goals:

    - Define Goals: Clearly define what you want to achieve with your new habits. For example, "I will exercise for 30 minutes every time I feel the urge to watch porn."
    - SMART Goals: Ensure your goals are Specific, Measurable, Achievable, Relevant, and Time-bound.[8]

4. Create a Routine:

    - Consistency: Establish a daily routine that incorporates your new habits. Consistency is key to forming new habits.
    - Schedule: Plan your day to include time for your new activities. For instance, if evening is a trigger time, schedule an activity like a workout session or a creative project during that time.

5. Use Positive Reinforcement:

    - Rewards: Reward yourself for sticking to your new habits. This could be something simple like enjoying a favorite treat or taking time for a relaxing activity.
    - Positive Feedback: Give yourself positive feedback for small wins and progress. This reinforces the new behavior.

6. Build a Support System:

   - Accountability: Share your goals with a trusted friend, family member, or support group. Regular check-ins can provide accountability.
   - Encouragement: Seek encouragement and support from those who understand your journey and can provide motivation.

7. Replace Negative Self-Talk:

   - Mindfulness: Practice mindfulness to stay aware of negative self-talk and replace it with positive affirmations.
   - Affirmations: Use positive affirmations to build self-esteem and reinforce your commitment to change.

8. Develop Stress Management Techniques:

   - Relaxation: Incorporate relaxation techniques such as deep breathing, yoga, or progressive muscle relaxation into your daily routine.
   - Healthy Outlets: Find healthy outlets for stress, such as physical activity, creative pursuits, or social interactions.

Benefits of New Habits

1. Breaking the Cycle:

   - Interrupt Patterns: New habits help interrupt the patterns that lead to porn consumption, making it easier to resist urges.
   - Reduced Triggers: Engaging in healthy activities can reduce the frequency and intensity of triggers.

2. Improved Mental Health:

   - Stress Reduction: Activities like exercise and mindfulness reduce stress and improve overall mental health.
   - Positive Emotions: Healthy habits can boost mood and create positive emotions, reducing the reliance on porn for emotional relief.

3. Enhanced Physical Health:

   - Fitness: Regular physical activity improves physical health, which can enhance overall well-being and self-esteem.
   - Energy Levels: Healthy habits increase energy levels, making it easier to stay motivated and engaged in daily life.

4. Stronger Relationships:

   - Social Connections: Engaging in social activities strengthens relationships and provides emotional support.
   - Communication Skills: Developing new habits can improve communication skills and deepen connections with others.

5. Increased Productivity:

   - Focus: Healthy habits improve focus and productivity, helping you achieve personal and professional goals.
   - Time Management: Better time management reduces idle time that might lead to porn consumption.

6. Building Self-Discipline:

   - Willpower: Establishing and maintaining new habits builds self-discipline and willpower, which are essential for long-term recovery.

- Resilience: Developing resilience through new habits makes it easier to handle setbacks and continue progressing.

Examples of New Habits

- Exercise Routine: Commit to a regular exercise routine, such as jogging, yoga, or weightlifting. Exercise releases endorphins, which improve mood and reduce stress.
- Creative Pursuits: Engage in creative activities like drawing, painting, writing, or playing a musical instrument. These activities provide a productive outlet for emotions.
- Reading and Learning: Replace time spent on porn with reading books, learning new skills, or taking online courses. This stimulates the mind and provides a sense of accomplishment.
- Social Activities: Join clubs, groups, or volunteer organizations to build social connections and create a sense of community.
- Mindfulness and Meditation: Practice mindfulness or meditation daily to increase self- awareness and reduce stress.

In conclusion, replacing bad habits with healthy ones is an effective strategy for overcoming porn addiction. By identifying triggers, choosing suitable alternatives, setting achievable goals, and maintaining consistency, porn addicts can create new, positive habits that support their recovery and lead to a healthier, more fulfilling life.[10]

1. Practice self-discipline: Strengthen self-discipline and self-control through consistent practice and effort. Learning to delay gratification and resist immediate impulses can help build resilience against addictive behaviors.
2. Celebrate successes and learn from setbacks: Acknowledge and celebrate achievements along the journey to recovery.

"Yes, I can quit."

Be compassionate with yourself in moments of relapse or setbacks, and use them as opportunities for learning and growth.

CHAPTER 6:
RELIGIONS AND DIVINE RELIGIONS

Many religions around the world emphasize the importance of moral conduct, particularly concerning sexual behavior and modesty. They often stress the need to lower one's gaze, avoid forbidden things, practice self-preservation, and maintain chastity. These principles are deeply embedded in the ethical and moral teachings of various faiths, guiding adherents to lead respectful and disciplined lives.

Lowering one's gaze is a common teaching across many religions. It involves avoiding looking at anything that might provoke lustful thoughts or inappropriate desires. This practice is seen as a way to maintain inner purity and respect for others. By controlling where they direct their attention, individuals can prevent their thoughts from straying into morally questionable areas. Avoiding forbidden things is another significant principle. Religions often define specific actions and behaviors as haram (forbidden) or sinful. These prohibitions include engaging in indecent behavior, consuming explicit material, or indulging in activities that lead to immorality. By steering clear of these forbidden actions, individuals are encouraged to live more virtuous and ethical lives.

Self-preservation is closely linked to the concept of avoiding sin and maintaining moral integrity.

It involves guarding one's soul and body against harmful influences and actions. This principle encourages individuals to practice self-control, remain vigilant against temptation, and uphold moral values. The emphasis on self-preservation helps individuals stay on a righteous path and avoid actions that could harm themselves or others.

Chastity, or maintaining sexual purity, is highly valued across many religious traditions. This principle often involves saving sexual relations for marriage and being faithful within that context. Premarital sex and adultery are typically condemned, and individuals are encouraged to practice sexual restraint. Chastity is seen as a means of preserving both spiritual and physical purity, promoting healthier relationships, and fostering a respectful society.

The principles of lowering one's gaze, avoiding forbidden things, self-preservation, and chastity are central to the moral teachings of many religions. These guidelines aim to help individuals lead disciplined and respectful lives, fostering a sense of inner purity and ethical behavior. By adhering to these principles, adherents are encouraged to live in a way that honors themselves, their relationships, and their broader communities.

Judaism

Judaism has comprehensive teachings on the topics of looking at taboos, sexual addiction, chastity, and morality. These teachings are rooted in the Torah, Talmud, and various rabbinic writings, emphasizing the importance of modesty, self-control, and ethical conduct.

Looking at Taboos and Sexual Addiction

Judaism places a strong emphasis on guarding one's eyes and thoughts from improper images and ideas. This principle is encapsulated in the concept of "Shmirat HaAinayim" (guarding the eyes). Jewish law discourages looking at anything that could lead to impure thoughts or actions, including pornography and other explicit materials.[1] The Talmud and other rabbinic texts stress the importance of avoiding situations that might provoke lustful thoughts or temptations.

Chastity and Morality

1. Chastity and Sexual Conduct: Judaism values sexual relations within the context of marriage and views them as a sacred act. Premarital and extramarital sexual relations are forbidden. The Torah outlines various laws related to sexual behavior, promoting chastity and fidelity. This helps maintain the sanctity of marriage and family life.
2. Modesty (Tzniut): Modesty is a fundamental value in Judaism, encompassing behavior, dress, and speech. Both men and women are encouraged to dress and behave in ways that reflect dignity and respect. This concept extends beyond physical appearance to include modesty in actions and interactions.
3. Self-Control and Purity: Judaism teaches the importance of self-discipline and control over one's desires. The laws of "Niddah" (family purity) regulate marital relations, emphasizing periods of separation and reunion to enhance marital sanctity and intimacy.
4. Ethical Conduct: Moral behavior in all aspects of life is a cornerstone of Jewish teaching. This includes honesty, integrity, and respect for others. Ethical conduct is seen as a reflection of one's relationship with God and adherence to His commandments.

Judaism's teachings on looking at taboos, sexual addiction, chastity, and morality are designed to promote a life of holiness, dignity, and ethical behavior. By guarding one's eyes, maintaining chastity, practicing modesty, and adhering to moral principles, individuals can live in accordance with Jewish values and contribute to a respectful and moral society. These teachings aim to foster healthy relationships, strong families, and a community built on respect and integrity.

Christianity

Christianity has clear and comprehensive teachings regarding looking at taboos, sexual addiction, chastity, and morality. These teachings are rooted in the Bible, particularly the New Testament, and are emphasized in the writings and teachings of church fathers, theologians, and contemporary Christian leaders.

Looking at Taboos and Sexual Addiction

Christianity strongly emphasizes the importance of purity in thought and deed. Jesus' teaching in the Sermon on the Mount states, "But I tell you that anyone who looks at a woman lustfully has already committed adultery with her in his heart" (Matthew 5:28). This highlights the significance of controlling one's thoughts and intentions. Christians are encouraged to avoid situations and materials that might lead to impure thoughts or actions, including pornography and other explicit content.[2]

Chastity and Morality

1. Chastity and Sexual Conduct: Christianity upholds sexual purity and reserves sexual relations for the context of marriage between a man and a woman. Premarital and extramarital sexual relations are considered sinful. The Bible teaches that the body is a temple of the Holy Spirit (1 Corinthians 6:19-20) and should be treated with respect and honor.
2. Modesty: Modesty in dress, speech, and behavior is highly valued in Christianity. Christians are called to present themselves in a manner that honors God and respects themselves and others. Modesty is seen as an outward expression of inner purity and integrity.
3. Self-Control and Purity: Self-control is a fruit of the Holy Spirit (Galatians 5:22-23) and is essential for maintaining purity. Christians are encouraged to flee from sexual immo-

rality and to pursue righteousness, faith, love, and peace (2 Timothy 2:22). Purity is not just about actions but also about maintaining a pure heart and mind.
4. Ethical Conduct: Christian ethics emphasize love, honesty, integrity, and respect for others. The teachings of Jesus, especially the command to "love your neighbor as yourself" (Mark 12:31), provide a foundation for moral behavior. Christians are called to live out their faith through actions that reflect their beliefs and uphold the moral standards set forth in the Bible.

Support and Accountability

Christianity emphasizes the importance of support and accountability within the community of believers. Christians are encouraged to confess their sins to one another and pray for each other for healing (James 5:16). This mutual support helps individuals struggling with sexual addiction to find strength and encouragement in their journey towards recovery. Churches often provide support groups and counseling to assist those battling addictions in breaking free and leading lives that align with Christian values. Redemption and Forgiveness

Central to Christian doctrine is the concept of redemption and forgiveness. Christianity teaches that no matter how deep one has fallen into sin, including sexual addiction, there is always hope for redemption through Jesus Christ. Repentance and seeking God's forgiveness are crucial steps towards healing and transformation. The Bible assures believers that if they confess their sins, God is faithful and just to forgive them and purify them from all unrighteousness (1 John 1:9).

Practical Steps for Overcoming Sexual Addiction

1. Spiritual Discipline: Engaging in regular spiritual practices such as prayer, meditation on scripture, and participation in worship services strengthens one's faith and resistance to

temptation. Developing a deep, personal relationship with God is foundational to overcoming addictions.

2. Mind Renewal: Christians are called to renew their minds through the truth of God's Word (Romans 12:2). By filling their minds with biblical teachings and positive, edifying content, they can counteract the negative influence of pornography and other sinful practices.

3. Healthy Relationships: Building and maintaining healthy, supportive relationships within the Christian community is crucial. These relationships provide accountability, encouragement, and practical help in resisting temptation and maintaining a lifestyle of purity.

Christianity offers a comprehensive framework for addressing issues related to looking at taboos, sexual addiction, chastity, and morality. Through its teachings, the faith promotes a life of purity, self-control, and ethical behavior, grounded in love and respect for others. The support of the Christian community, along with the principles of redemption and forgiveness, provides a path to recovery and a life that reflects Christian values. By adhering to these teachings, Christians seek to honor God and contribute to a society that upholds dignity and moral integrity.

Islam

Prophet Muhammad (peace be upon him) provided clear guidance on the importance of lowering one's gaze to maintain purity of heart and avoid sinful thoughts and actions. This principle is emphasized in both the Quran and the Hadith (the sayings and actions of the Prophet). Here are some key teachings and examples from the life of the Prophet Muhammad regarding lowering one's gaze:

Quranic Foundation

The Quran explicitly instructs both men and women to lower their gaze as a means of guarding their modesty[11]:

- For Men:

    "Tell the believing men to lower their gaze and guard their private parts; that is purer for them. Indeed, Allah is Acquainted with what they do." (Quran 24:30)

- For Women:

    "And tell the believing women to lower their gaze and guard their private parts and not expose their adornment except that which [necessarily] appears thereof..." (Quran 24:31)

These verses set the foundation for the practice of lowering one's gaze to avoid improper thoughts and maintain moral integrity.

Hadith on Lowering One's Gaze

Prophet Muhammad elaborated on this principle through various Hadith, providing practical advice and examples for his followers[12]:

1. Avoiding the Second Glance:

    The Prophet said: "Do not follow a (forbidden) glance with another one. The first is permitted for you but not the second." (Jami` at-Tirmidhi 2777) This Hadith indicates that an accidental first glance is forgiven, but deliberately looking again is not permissible, emphasizing self-control and immediate correction.

2. Controlling the Eyes to Guard the Heart:

The Prophet Muhammad stated: "The eyes are the lustful arrows of Satan. Whoever lowers his gaze for Allah, He will bestow upon him a refreshing sweetness which he will find in his heart on the day he meets Him." (Al-Mustadrak Al-Hakim 7875) This saying highlights the spiritual reward of lowering one's gaze and the inner peace it brings to a believer.

3. Eyes as the Gateway to the Heart:

In another Hadith, the Prophet said: "The glance is a poisoned arrow of Satan. Whoever lowers his gaze from looking at the beauties of women (or men), Allah will place in his heart the sweetness of faith, the taste of which he will experience." (Ibn Majah 4171) This reinforces the idea that controlling one's gaze is essential for protecting the heart from sinful desires and fostering a deep, fulfilling faith.[3]

Examples from the Life of the Prophet Muhammad

1. Incident of the Companion Jareer ibn Abdullah:

Jareer ibn Abdullah narrated an incident where he asked the Prophet Muhammad about an accidental glance at a woman. The Prophet advised him to immediately avert his gaze: "Jareer ibn Abdullah said: I asked the Messenger of Allah about an accidental glance (at a woman). He commanded me to avert my gaze." (Sahih Muslim 2159) This example demonstrates the practical application of the principle of lowering one's gaze.

2. Admonition to Fadl ibn Abbas:

-During the Farewell Pilgrimage, Al-Fadl ibn Abbas was riding behind the Prophet when a beautiful woman from the Khath'am tribe approached to ask a question. Al-Fadl began to stare at her, so the Prophet gently turned his face away:

"Al-Fadl bin 'Abbas was riding behind the Messenger of Allah and a woman from Khath'am came asking the Prophet for a religious verdict. Al-Fadl started looking at her as she was beautiful. The Prophet turned Al-Fadl's face to the other side." (Sahih al-Bukhari 1513) This incident shows the Prophet's practical intervention to help his companions maintain Their behaver in self-control.

Chastity in Sex

Quranic Teachings:

Chastity is highly valued in Islam, and maintaining sexual purity is considered essential for spiritual and moral well-being. The Quran emphasizes the importance of chastity and fidelity within marriage.

- "And those who guard their private parts except from their wives or those their right hands possess, for indeed, they will not be blamed. But whoever seeks beyond that, then those are the transgressors." (Quran 23:5-7) This verse underscores that sexual relations are permissible only within the confines of marriage, and any sexual activity outside of marriage is considered a transgression.

Hadith Teachings:

The Hadith also provide clear guidance on the importance of chastity and the need to avoid situations that may lead to sinful behavior.

The Prophet Muhammad (peace be upon him) said, "Whoever can guarantee (the chastity of) what is between his jaws (i.e., his tongue) and what is between his legs (i.e., his private parts), I guarantee Paradise for him." (Sahih al-Bukhari) This Hadith highlights the significance of controlling one's speech and sexual behavior as keys to attaining Paradise.

The Story of Prophet Yusuf (Joseph) in Islam

The story of Prophet Yusuf (Joseph) in Islam is a profound example of chastity, integrity, and the importance of lowering one's gaze. This narrative, detailed in Surah Yusuf (Chapter 12) of the Quran, highlights the trials and virtues of Yusuf, who is revered for his unwavering faith and moral fortitude.

Yusuf, the son of Prophet Yaqub (Jacob), was known for his exceptional beauty and righteousness. His brothers, driven by jealousy, plotted against him. Yusuf had a dream in which he saw eleven stars, the sun, and the moon prostrating to him. When he shared this dream with his father, Yaqub recognized its significance and cautioned Yusuf not to disclose it to his brothers, fearing their jealousy. Nevertheless, their envy led them to cast Yusuf into a well, falsely telling their father that a wolf had devoured him. Yusuf was later found by a passing caravan and sold into slavery. He was taken to Egypt, where he was sold to a high-ranking official referred to as Al-Aziz.

In Egypt, Yusuf was placed in the household of Al-Aziz. As Yusuf grew older, his good looks and noble character attracted the attention of Zulaikha, the wife of Al-Aziz. She attempted to seduce Yusuf, but he remained steadfast in his faith and commitment to chastity. The Quran describes this moment: "And she, in whose house he was, sought to seduce him. She closed the doors and said, 'Come, you.' He said, 'I seek refuge in Allah. Indeed, He is my master, who has made good my residence. Indeed, wrongdoers will not succeed.'" (Quran 12:23). Yusuf's immediate reaction was to seek refuge in Allah, demonstrating his fear of God and his commitment to moral integrity.

Despite the temptation and difficult circumstances, Yusuf chose to uphold his chastity and honor. The Quran further states: "And she certainly determined to seduce him, and he would have inclined to her had he not seen the proof of his Lord. And thus [it was] that We should avert from him evil and immorality. Indeed, he was of Our chosen servants." (Quran 12:24). Yusuf's ability to resist temptation was bolstered by his faith and his awareness of Allah's presence, which helped him remain chaste and righteous.

When Zulaikha's advances were rejected, she accused Yusuf of attempting to assault her. To prove his innocence, a witness suggested that if Yusuf's shirt was torn from the back, it would indicate he was fleeing from her, but if torn from the front, it would imply he was attacking her. Yusuf's shirt was found torn from the back, confirming his innocence. Nevertheless, to avoid scandal, Al-Aziz decided to imprison Yusuf. Even in the face of false accusations and injustice, Yusuf remained patient and faithful to Allah.

While in prison, Yusuf's gift of dream interpretation became known. He accurately interpreted the dreams of two fellow prisoners, one who would be restored to his position and the other who would be executed. His ability became renowned, and later, when the Pharaoh had a troubling dream that none could interpret, Yusuf was called upon. He interpreted the Pharaoh's dream, predicting seven years of plentiful harvests followed by seven years of severe famine, advising on how to prepare for the impending hardship. Impressed by his wisdom, the Pharaoh released Yusuf and appointed him to a high position of authority, overseeing the granaries of Egypt.

During the famine, Yusuf's brothers came to Egypt seeking food, not recognizing him. Yusuf tested them by accusing them of being spies and eventually revealed his identity, forgiving them for their past actions. He invited his family to settle in Egypt, thus reuniting with his father, Yaqub.

The story of Prophet Yusuf serves as an enduring lesson in chastity and the importance of lowering one's gaze. Yusuf's unwavering faith in Allah helped him overcome severe trials and temptations. His reliance on God's guidance and protection was the cornerstone of his moral integrity. Despite being in a vulnerable situation, Yusuf maintained his chastity. His ability to resist temptation and uphold his principles is a powerful example for all believers. Yusuf's life story teaches the importance of patience and perseverance in the face of hardship and injustice. His eventual vindication underscores the belief that Allah supports those who remain steadfast in their faith. The story emphasizes the value of moral integrity and the importance of making righteous choices, even when faced with significant pressure and temptation.

Ali Ibn Abi Talib

Imam Ali ibn Abi Talib, the fourth Caliph of Islam and a cousin and son-in-law of Prophet Muhammad (peace be upon him), is highly revered in Islamic tradition for his wisdom, piety, and eloquence. Numerous sayings and teachings attributed to him emphasize the importance of chastity, moral conduct, and the virtue of guarding one's gaze.

Chastity and Guarding the Gaze

1. On Chastity:

    Imam Ali often spoke about the virtues of chastity and self-control. He emphasized that maintaining chastity is a key component of piety and moral integrity. One of his well-known sayings is:

    - "Chastity is the ornament of both men and women."

    This highlights that chastity is a noble quality that enhances the dignity and honor of individuals, regardless of their gender.

2. On Guarding the Gaze:

    Imam Ali also stressed the importance of lowering one's gaze to avoid immoral thoughts and actions. He taught that controlling one's vision is a crucial aspect of maintaining personal purity and righteousness. A notable saying attributed to him is:

- "The eyes are the scouts of the heart, and the heart is the fortress. Therefore, lower your gaze, and it will guard your heart and chastity."

This saying underscores the idea that what one sees can influence the heart and lead to either purity or corruption. By lowering the gaze, a person protects their heart from sinful desires and maintains their chastity.

3. Avoiding Temptation:

   Imam Ali advised against exposing oneself to situations that could lead to temptation and sin. He believed in proactive measures to safeguard one's morality and spiritual well-being. Another of his sayings includes:

- "The one who gazes frequently at the beauty of others' women, his heart becomes blind." This emphasizes that frequent indulgence in looking at forbidden things can dull one's moral and spiritual senses, leading to a loss of inner sight and guidance.

Example of Imam Ali's Teachings in Practice

Imam Ali's own life serves as a testament to his teachings on chastity and guarding the gaze. He was known for his deep piety and adherence to Islamic principles. His conduct set a high standard for Muslims to follow:

- Incident of the Conquered City:

It is narrated that during one of the battles, after the victory, when the Muslim soldiers entered the city, Imam Ali instructed them to maintain their moral conduct and avoid looking at women or engaging in any behavior that could lead to moral corruption. This act was to ensure that the soldiers did not succumb to any form of temptation and maintained their chastity and honor.

Hinduism

Hinduism emphasizes living a virtuous and spiritually fulfilling life, guided by the principles of dharma (moral duty), karma (actions and their consequences), and self-control.

Pornography and Sensory Control

Hindu teachings stress the importance of controlling the senses and avoiding actions that lead to moral and spiritual decline. The concept of "Brahmacharya," which means celibacy or self-discipline, is particularly valued for students and spiritual aspirants. Engaging with pornography is considered harmful to one's spiritual journey and moral integrity. Ancient texts like the Manusmriti highlight the need to maintain purity in thoughts and actions.

Chastity and Moral Values

Chastity, or Brahmacharya, is seen as crucial for spiritual purity and reaching higher states of consciousness. Hindu scriptures such as the Bhagavad Gita emphasize leading a life of virtue, which includes sexual purity and fidelity within marriage. While the pursuit of pleasure (Kama) is acknowledged, it should always align with dharma and be confined to the context of marriage and procreation.[4]

Buddhism

Buddhism focuses on the path to enlightenment through ethical living, mental discipline, and wisdom. The teachings of the Buddha provide a framework for leading a moral life that avoids harm to oneself and others.

Pornography: Buddhism teaches the importance of right conduct (sila), which includes abstaining from sexual misconduct. The Noble Eightfold Path, which guides Buddhists toward enlightenment, includes Right Action, which involves avoiding actions that cause harm, including indulging in pornography. Mindfulness (sati) helps individuals be aware of their thoughts and actions, promoting self-control and avoiding harmful behaviors.

Chastity and Morals: Monks and nuns take vows of celibacy, dedicating their lives to spiritual practice without the distractions of sexual activity. Lay Buddhists are encouraged to practice sexual restraint and fidelity within marriage. The Five Precepts, which lay Buddhists follow, include refraining from sexual misconduct, defined as any sexual behavior that causes harm or suffering to oneself or others. Maintaining purity of mind and reducing suffering caused by attachment and desire are central to Buddhist ethics.[5]

Sikhism

Sikhism, founded by Guru Nanak in the 15th century, emphasizes living a truthful and honest life while being mindful of one's actions. The teachings of the Gurus provide a moral compass for Sikhs to follow.

Pornography and Blindness: Sikh teachings discourage indulgence in activities that lead to moral corruption. Guru Granth Sahib, the central religious scripture, emphasizes living a life of virtue, self-control, and purity. Engaging in pornography is seen as contrary to these principles. The Sikh Rehat Maryada (Sikh code of conduct) encourages Sikhs to maintain purity in thought and action.

Chastity and Morals: Sikhs are encouraged to live a life of high moral standards, which includes being faithful in marriage and maintaining sexual purity. The concept of "Kaam" (lust) is one of the five thieves (vices) that Sikhs strive to overcome to achieve spiritual growth.[6]

Chastity before marriage and fidelity within marriage are important virtues, reflecting the commitment to living a righteous life.

Sabian-Mandaean

The Sabian-Mandaean religion is an ancient Gnostic faith with a focus on purity, rituals, and adherence to moral principles. Its teachings emphasize the importance of maintaining spiritual and physical cleanliness.

Pornography: Mandaeans emphasize purity and avoiding actions that defile the soul. Viewing pornography would be considered impure and against the principles of maintaining spiritual cleanliness. The religion's rituals and teachings stress the importance of avoiding sinful behaviors and focusing on spiritual purity.[7]

Chastity and Morals: Chastity is important in Mandaean teachings, with an emphasis on leading a pure and righteous life. Sexual relations are to be kept within the bounds of marriage, and moral conduct is highly valued. The Mandaean texts provide guidance on maintaining ethical behavior and purity.

Other Religions

Other religions also provide guidelines regarding moral conduct, chastity, and avoiding harmful behaviors.

Zoroastrianism: This ancient religion emphasizes the duality of good and evil. Followers are encouraged to lead lives of purity and righteousness. Sexual purity and fidelity are highly valued, and behaviors like consuming pornography would be discouraged as they align with deceit and impurity. The Avesta, the sacred Zoroastrian texts, outline the importance of maintaining moral integrity.[8]

Jainism: Jainism advocates for strict ethical principles, including non-violence (ahimsa), truthfulness, and celibacy for monks and nuns. Lay Jains are also encouraged to practice sexual restraint and maintain purity in thoughts and actions.[9] The teachings of Mahavira, the 24th Tirthankara, emphasize the importance of leading a life of self-discipline and ethical conduct.

Bahá'í Faith: The Bahá'í teachings emphasize moral conduct, chastity before marriage, and fidelity within marriage. Engaging in pornography is viewed as harmful to both spiritual and moral development. The writings of Bahá'u'lláh, the founder of the Bahá'í Faith, stress the importance of leading a life that reflects divine virtues and purity.[10]

Across these various religions, there is a common thread emphasizing the importance of moral conduct, self-control, and purity. Pornography is generally seen as detrimental to one's spiritual and moral well-being. Chastity and maintaining high ethical standards are valued, and individuals are encouraged to lead lives that reflect these principles. These teachings aim to foster healthy relationships, personal integrity, and spiritual growth. By adhering to these moral guidelines, adherents of these faiths strive to live in a way that honors their spiritual commitments and contributes to a respectful and moral society.

SUMMARY OF "SMILE, YOU ARE ADDICTED"

In "Smile, You Are Addicted," I aim to offer heartfelt advice and guidance to the current and future generations. This book is born out of my deep concern for the moral and emotional well-being of our society, particularly as I witness the widespread corruption and disintegration of families due to the deceptive allure of pornography.

The title, "Smile, You Are Addicted," was chosen deliberately to start with a positive word, "smile," followed by "addicted," to make the reader aware and self-admit the reality of their addiction. This juxtaposition is meant to gently confront the reader with the truth of their situation, encouraging them to face their addiction head-on and seek recovery. The tone throughout the book is light and engaging, designed to make the difficult subject matter more approachable and less intimidating for the reader.

I have observed how pornography, with its false promises and harmful content, has ensnared many of my loved ones, friends, and acquaintances. Some have seen their families fall apart and now suffer from profound anxiety and distress. It is this personal connection to the victims of pornography that has compelled me to write this book. I see it as both a human and moral duty to share my insights and provide a path to recovery and healing.

The book is written with an emotional, loving, and compassionate tone, aiming to be a balm and healing medicine for those who are struggling. Through my words, I hope to reach the hearts and minds of those affected, offering them comfort and practical advice to break free from the grip of addiction.

In "Smile, You Are Addicted," I explore the deceptive nature of pornography and its destructive impact on individuals and families. I provide real-life examples and stories of those who have overcome addiction, highlighting the strength and resilience needed to reclaim one's life. I offer strategies for self-awareness, goal setting, and the development of new, healthier habits to replace the harmful ones.

This book is not just a collection of advice, but a call to action to recognize the dangers of pornography, reclaim one's life, and restore the health and unity of our families and communities. By addressing these issues with empathy and understanding, I hope to foster a better future where individuals can thrive in an environment of love, respect, and integrity.

Ultimately, "Smile, You Are Addicted" is about transformation and hope. It is a guide to help readers confront their addiction with honesty, embrace the process of recovery with positivity, and rebuild their lives with strength and dignity. Through this book, I aspire to be a source of support and inspiration, helping readers to navigate their journey towards a healthier and more fulfilling life.

SOURCES

Chapter 1

1. Historical Context and Roles of Women:

   - **Source: Bock, Gisela. *Women in European History*. Blackwell Publishing, 2002.**

     - **Attribution:** "In bygone eras, women were shielded from the harsh realities of financial responsibility, their duties centered squarely on the hearth and home".

2. Economic and Social Upheaval:

   - **Source: Avakian, Arlene Voski, and Barbara Haber, eds. *From Betty Crocker to Feminist Food Studies: Critical Perspectives on Women and Food*. University of Massachusetts Press, 2005.**

     - **Attribution:** "Wars ravaged nations, famines struck with merciless force, and deadly diseases stalked the land, leaving devastation in their wake".

3. Impact of the Industrial Revolution:

   - **Source: Collins, Gail. *The Industrial Revolution and the Changing Role of Women in Society*. Oxford University Press, 2009.**

- **Attribution:** "The industrial revolution, with its promise of progress and prosperity, proved to be a double-edged sword for women".

4. Economic Participation:

- **Source: Hoffman, Saul D., and Susan Averett. *Women and the Economy: Family, Work, and Pay*. Pearson, 2015.**

  - **Attribution:** "As they entered factories and mills, they gradually drifted from their fundamental responsibilities, leaving a void in the fabric of family life".

5. Modern Impacts and Social Changes:

- **Source: Hochschild, Arlie Russell, and Anne Machung. *The Second Shift: Working Families and the Revolution at Home*. Penguin Books, 2012.**

  - **Attribution:** "Divorce rates soared, and the ranks of single mothers swelled, bearing witness to the fraying of familial bonds and the erosion of societal norms".

6. Social and Cultural Impact:

- **Source: Ryan, Barbara. *Feminism and the Women's Movement: Dynamics of Change in Social Movement Ideology and Activism*. Routledge, 1992.**

  - **Attribution:** "With the rise of industrialization came a stark realization: the traditional roles of women as caregivers and homemakers were no longer sustainable".

Chapter 2

Historical Access to Pornography:

1. **Source**: Dines, Gail. *Pornland: How Porn Has Hijacked Our Sexuality*. Beacon Press, 2010.

    - **Attribution**: "In the not-so-distant past, access to pornographic material was largely confined to paper publications or videos, typically relegated to discreet adult-only spaces".

Impact of the Internet on Pornography:

2. **Source**: Paul, Pamela. *Pornified: How Pornography Is Damaging Our Lives, Our Relationships, and Our Families*. Times Books, 2005.

    - **Attribution**: "With the rise of computer programming and the proliferation of the World Wide Web, pornographic material became just a click away for anyone with an internet connection".

3. **Source**: Cooper, Al, et al. *Cybersex: The Impact of the Internet on Sexuality*. Routledge, 2000.

    - **Attribution**: "The anonymity and convenience offered by online platforms shattered the barriers that once confined pornography to the shadows".

Consequences of Internet Pornography:

4. **Source**: Eberstadt, Mary. *Adam and Eve after the Pill: Paradoxes of the Sexual Revolution*. Ignatius Press, 2012.

    - **Attribution**: "Suddenly, society found itself inundated with a deluge of explicit content, bombarding unsuspecting users with images and videos that were previously confined to the fringes of society".

5. **Source**: Zillmann, Dolf, and Bryant, Jennings. *Pornography: Research Advances and Policy Considerations*. Routledge, 1989.

    - **Attribution**: "As access to pornography became ubiquitous, a new generation emerged, characterized by a distorted understanding of sexuality and intimacy".

6. **Source**: Malamuth, Neil M., and Edward Donnerstein. *Pornography and Sexual Aggression*. Academic Press, 1984.

    - **Attribution**: "The cultural landscape underwent a tectonic shift, as traditional values and norms gave way to a brave new world of instant gratification and moral relativism".

Psychological and Social Impact:

7. **Source**: Layden, Mary Anne. *The Social Costs of Pornography: A Collection of Papers*. Witherspoon Institute, 2010.

    - **Attribution**: "As we confront the legacy of this digital revolution, we must reckon with the profound impact of pornography on our collective psyche".

8. **Source**: Manning, Jimmie, et al. *Internet Pornography: Assessing the Impact on Relationships and Well-being*. Nova Science Publishers, 2016.

    - **Attribution**: "As access to pornography became ubiquitous, a new generation emerged, characterized by a distorted understanding of sexuality and intimacy".

Chapter 3

The Brain and Its Wondrous Network:

1. **Source**: Doidge, Norman. *The Brain That Changes Itself: Stories of Personal Triumph from the Frontiers of Brain Science.* Viking Penguin, 2007.

    - **Attribution**: "At the very core of our being lies the brain, a masterful creation that serves as the command center of our bodies and minds".

2. **Source**: Kandel, Eric R. *In Search of Memory: The Emergence of a New Science of Mind.* W. W. Norton & Company, 2006.

    - **Attribution**: "Within its vast expanse, billions of neurons fire and connect, forming intricate pathways that shape our experiences and shape our understanding of the world".

Interaction with Hormones:

3. **Source**: Sapolsky, Robert M. *Why Zebras Don't Get Ulcers: The Acclaimed Guide to Stress, Stress- Related Diseases, and Coping.* Holt Paperbacks, 2004.

    - **Attribution**: "The brain's interaction with hormones is a complex and intricate dance that regulates a wide array of bodily functions, emotions, and behaviors".

4. **Source**: McEwen, Bruce S. *The End of Stress As We Know It.* Dana Press, 2002.

    - **Attribution**: "For example, when the body experiences stress, the hypothalamus signals the pituitary gland to release adrenocorticotropic hormone (ACTH), which stimulates the adrenal glands to release cortisol, the body's primary stress hormone".

Dopamine and Addiction:

5. **Source**: Volkow, Nora D., and Ting-Kai Li. *Drug Addiction: The Neurobiology of Behaviour Gone Awry*. Nature Reviews Neuroscience, 2004.

    - **Attribution**: "Dopamine is a neurotransmitter—a chemical messenger in the brain—that plays a key role in reward-motivated behavior, pleasure, and reinforcement learning".

6. **Source**: Nestler, Eric J. *Is There a Common Molecular Pathway for Addiction?*. Nature Neuroscience, 2005.

    - **Attribution**: "However, with repeated exposure to highly stimulating activities, such as excessive pornography use, the brain's reward system can become dysregulated".

Testosterone and Its Effects:

7. **Source**: Bancroft, John. *Human Sexuality and Its Problems*. Elsevier Health Sciences, 2009.

    - **Attribution**: "Testosterone is a hormone primarily produced in the testicles in males and in smaller amounts in the ovaries in females. It plays a crucial role in the development of male reproductive tissues, as well as promoting secondary sexual characteristics".

8. **Source**: Gray, Peter B., et al. *Human Male Testosterone, Pair Bonding and Fatherhood*. Endocrine Reviews, 2002.

    - **Attribution**: "Some research suggests that excessive pornography use may lead to desensitization of the brain's reward system, including the hypothalamic-pituitary- gonadal (HPG) axis, which regulates testosterone production".

Psychological Health and Addiction:

9. **Source**: Carnes, Patrick. *Out of the Shadows: Understanding Sexual Addiction.* Hazelden Publishing, 2001.

    - **Attribution**: "The allure of pornography can be intoxicating, drawing individuals into a seemingly endless cycle of consumption with devastating consequences for their mental well-being and sense of self-worth".

10. **Source**: Wilson, Gary, and Paula Hall. *Your Brain on Porn: Internet Pornography and the Emerging Science of Addiction.* Commonwealth Publishing, 2014.

    - **Attribution**: "As addiction takes hold, the consequences become increasingly dire. Mental health deteriorates, as individuals struggle with feelings of shame, guilt, and worthlessness".

11. Published on Al Jazeera.net on 7/18/2018, Written by Ibrahim Al-Sayed

Chapter 4

Victims of Pornography - From Young to Old, Women to Men Exploitation of Young People:

1. **Source**: "Internet Pornography and Adolescents: The Cognitive and Emotional Consequences" by Elizabeth K. Englander

    - **Details**: This study explores how exposure to pornography during adolescence can distort perceptions of sex and relationships, leading to unrealistic expectations and unhealthy attitudes.

Exploitation of Women:

2. **Source**: "Pornography and Sexual Violence: A New Look at the Research" by Neil Malamuth and Mary Koss

   - **Details**: This research highlights how women are objectified and dehumanized in pornography, affecting their dignity and humanity.

Impact on Men:

3. **Source**: "The Impact of Internet Pornography on Men: A Review of Research" by Paul J. Wright

   - **Details**: This review discusses how men can become addicted to pornography, leading to a cycle of shame, relationship issues, and self-worth problems.

Exploitation of the Elderly:

4. **Source**: "Elder Abuse and Exploitation: Pornography's Impact" by the National Center on Elder Abuse

   - **Details**: This report examines cases of elder abuse in nursing homes and assisted living facilities, including exploitation through pornography.

Lily's Story

Pornography Addiction and Personal Stories:

5. **Source**: "Treating Pornography Addiction: The Essential Tools for Recovery" by Kevin B. Skinner

   - **Details**: This book provides detailed personal stories and case studies of individuals like Lily who have strug-

gled with pornography addiction and their journey towards recovery.
- **Link**: Treating Pornography Addiction

The Impact

Impact on Women:

6. **Source**: "The Social Costs of Pornography: A Collection of Papers" by Mary Anne Layden

    - **Details**: This collection discusses how unrealistic portrayals in pornography affect women's self-esteem, body image, and relationships.

Impact on Men:

7. **Source**: "Pornography Consumption and Erectile Dysfunction: A Review" by Gert Martin Hald

    - **Details**: This review explores how pornography consumption can lead to erectile dysfunction, reduced libido, and difficulty forming genuine connections.

Societal Level Impact:

8. **Source**: "Pornography and Public Health: Understanding the Impact and Preparing for a Response" by Gail Dines

    - **Details**: This article discusses how pornography shapes societal attitudes towards sex, relationships, and gender roles, and its broader impact on public health and social services.

The Industry

Economic and Global Reach:

9. **Source**: "The Economics of Adult Entertainment" by Benjamin Edelman

    - **Details**: This study examines the revenue streams, global reach, and economic impact of the pornography industry.

Technological Advancements:

10. **Source**: "The Role of Technology in the Expansion of the Pornography Industry" by Peter Johnson

    - **Details**: This article discusses how technological innovations, such as streaming services and virtual reality, have revolutionized the pornography industry.

The Art and Artists of the Porn Industry

Jewish Influence:

11. **Source**: "Jews and the American Pornography Industry" by Nathan Abrams

    - **Details**: This research explores the historical and cultural influence of Jewish individuals in the development and growth of the American pornography industry.

12. **Source:** "article - aljazeera.net 18/7/2018 ibrahim assayed"

Chapter 5

Free Will and Overcoming Addiction:

1. **Source**: Baumeister, Roy F., and John Tierney. *Willpower: Rediscovering the Greatest Human Strength*. Penguin Books, 2011.

    - **Attribution**: "Human free will refers to the capacity of individuals to make choices and decisions without being determined by external factors or forces".

2. **Source**: Vohs, Kathleen D., and Roy F. Baumeister. *Handbook of Self-Regulation: Research, Theory, and Applications*. Guilford Press, 2011.

    - **Attribution**: "Overcoming addiction to pornography requires harnessing this free will to initiate and sustain change".

Self-Awareness in Recovery:

3. **Source**: Tolle, Eckhart. *The Power of Now: A Guide to Spiritual Enlightenment*. New World Library, 1997.

    - **Attribution**: "Self-awareness is a crucial component in the recovery from porn addiction. It involves recognizing and understanding one's thoughts, emotions, and behaviors related to pornography use".

4. **Source**: Brown, Brené. *Daring Greatly: How the Courage to Be Vulnerable Transforms the Way We Live, Love, Parent, and Lead*. Gotham Books, 2012.

    - **Attribution**: "By becoming more self-aware, individuals can identify the underlying causes and triggers of their addiction, which is essential for effective recovery".

Seeking and Receiving Help:

5. **Source**: Miller, William R., and Stephen Rollnick. *Motivational Interviewing: Helping People Change*. Guilford Press, 2012.

    - **Attribution**: "Seeking and receiving help is highly effective for individuals struggling with porn addiction. The process of reaching out for support and accepting assistance can provide crucial resources, guidance, and encouragement".

6. **Source**: Carnes, Patrick. *Out of the Shadows: Understanding Sexual Addiction*. Hazelden Publishing, 2001.

    - **Attribution**: "Professional therapists and counselors who specialize in addiction can provide evidence-based treatment methods, such as Cognitive Behavioral Therapy (CBT), which helps individuals change their thinking patterns and behaviors related to pornography use".

Setting Goals for Recovery:

7. **Source**: Locke, Edwin A., and Gary P. Latham. *A Theory of Goal Setting and Task Performance*. Prentice-Hall, 1990.

    - **Attribution**: "Setting goals for recovery is a crucial strategy for porn addicts aiming to overcome their addiction. Establishing clear, achievable goals provides direction, motivation, and a sense of purpose".

8. **Source**: Dweck, Carol S. *Mindset: The New Psychology of Success*. Ballantine Books, 2006.

    - **Attribution**: "By setting specific, measurable, achievable, relevant, and time-bound (SMART) goals, individuals can create a structured path towards recovery and track their progress effectively".

Creating New Habits to Replace Bad Habits:

9. **Source**: Clear, James. *Atomic Habits: An Easy & Proven Way to Build Good Habits & Break Bad Ones*. Avery, 2018.

    - **Attribution**: "Creating new habits to replace the bad habit of porn consumption is an essential strategy for reducing addiction. This involves identifying triggers, choosing healthier alternatives, and consistently practicing these new behaviors until they become ingrained".

10. **Source**: Duhigg, Charles. *The Power of Habit: Why We Do What We Do in Life and Business*. Random House, 2012.

    - **Attribution**: "By focusing on small, incremental changes and celebrating progress, individuals can build new, positive habits that support their recovery and lead to a healthier, more fulfilling life".

Lowering One's Gaze and Chastity:

11. **Source**: Nasr, Seyyed Hossein. *The Study Quran: A New Translation and Commentary*. HarperOne, 2015.

    - **Attribution**: "The Quran explicitly instructs both men and women to lower their gaze as a means of guarding their modesty".

12. **Source**: Al-Bukhari, Muhammad ibn Ismail. *Sahih al-Bukhari*. Darussalam Publishers, 1997.

    - **Attribution**: "The Prophet Muhammad elaborated on this principle through various Hadith, providing practical advice and examples for his followers".

Chapter 6

Religions and divine religions

1. **Judaism:** Teachings on guarding one's eyes and thoughts from improper images and ideas can be found in the Talmud and various rabbinic texts.

   - "Shmirat HaAinayim" (guarding the eyes): Discussed extensively in Jewish law and rabbinic literature.
   - **Talmud**: Emphasis on avoiding situations that might provoke lustful thoughts or temptations.

2. **Christianity**: Teachings on purity in thought and deed are rooted in the Bible, particularly the New Testament.

   - Matthew 5:28: Jesus' teaching on lustful thoughts.
   - 1 Corinthians 6:19-20: The body as a temple of the Holy Spirit.
   - Galatians 5:22-23: Self-control as a fruit of the Holy Spirit.
   - Mark 12:31: The command to "love your neighbor as yourself."
   - James 5:16: Confessing sins and praying for each other.
   - 1 John 1:9: Assurance of God's forgiveness.

3. **Islam**: Guidance on lowering one's gaze and maintaining purity is found in the Quran and Hadith.

   - Quran 24:30-31: Instructions for men and women to lower their gaze.
   - **Hadith**: Various sayings of Prophet Muhammad on controlling the gaze and maintaining chastity.
   - Example from Prophet Yusuf's story: Detailed in Surah Yusuf (Chapter 12) of the Quran.

4. **Hinduism**: Emphasis on controlling the senses and maintaining chastity is rooted in ancient texts.

    - **Manusmriti**: Highlights the need for purity in thoughts and actions.
    - **Bhagavad Gita**: Emphasis on leading a life of virtue and sexual purity.

5. **Buddhism**: Teachings on ethical living and avoiding sexual misconduct are part of the Noble Eightfold Path.

    - **Right Action**: Involves avoiding actions that cause harm, including indulging in pornography.
    - **Five Precepts**: Refraining from sexual misconduct.

6. **Sikhism**: Teachings on moral conduct and purity are emphasized in Guru Granth Sahib and the Sikh Rehat Maryada.

    - **Guru Granth Sahib**: Central religious scripture emphasizing virtue and self-control.
    - **Sikh Rehat Maryada**: Encourages maintaining purity in thought and action.

7. **Sabian-Mandaean**: Emphasis on purity and avoiding actions that defile the soul.

    - **Mandaean texts**: Guidance on maintaining ethical behavior and purity.

8. **Zoroastrianism**: Emphasis on purity and righteousness in the Avesta.

    - **Avesta**: Sacred texts outlining the importance of maintaining moral integrity.

9. **Jainism**: Advocates for strict ethical principles and celibacy for monks and nuns.

- **Teachings of Mahavira**: Emphasis on self-discipline and ethical conduct.

10. **Bahá'í Faith**: Emphasis on moral conduct and chastity in the writings of Bahá'u'lláh.

    - **Writings of Bahá'u'lláh**: Stress the importance of leading a life that reflects divine virtues and purity.

AUTHOR

Born in April 1982 in Najaf, Iraq, the author has always harbored a deep interest in writing and producing journalism, particularly using modern computer technologies. The journey into the world of journalism and media production began after completing studies in nursing. While nursing was a fulfilling field, the author discovered a deeper passion and love for journalistic production, writing, and contributing to society's effectiveness and productivity.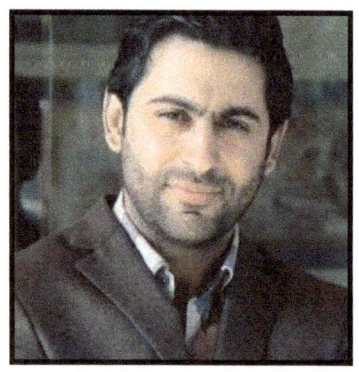

Recognizing this newfound passion, the author furthered education at the Union Center for Media Training Institute in Lebanon, earning a certificate in journalistic production. This education laid the foundation for a successful career in media.

The author's career in media blossomed with the role of head of the media department in one of Iraq's governorates. Leadership skills and editorial expertise were showcased in supervising the editorship of a prominent magazine. Through these roles, significant contributions have been made to the field of journalism, blending a healthcare background with media acumen to provide insightful, well-rounded content.

In addition to his journalism career, the author has taught graphics for more than 1,000 hours, successfully graduating dozens of students from his training courses. His dedication to education extended to teaching computer skills to newcomers in Canada at Medicine Hat College in Brooks, Alberta, providing them with essential tools for integration and success in their new environment.

The author would like to extend heartfelt thanks to his wonderful wife, who holds a master's degree in behavioral analysis. Her distinguished comments, academic analytical outlook, and immense interest in the family have been invaluable in helping complete this book. Her care, patience, and unwavering support have provided a nurturing environment for their little boy and have been a constant source of inspiration and pride throughout this journey.

Author: Montazar Alkefaae
Translated by: Haider Al-Ankushi
Edited by: Qasim Al-kefaae & Ai
Design: HMDPUBLISHING